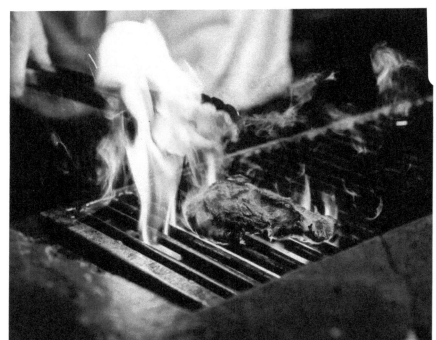

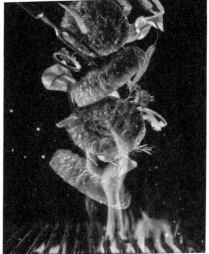

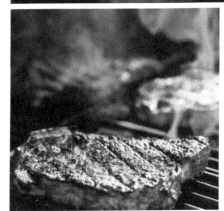

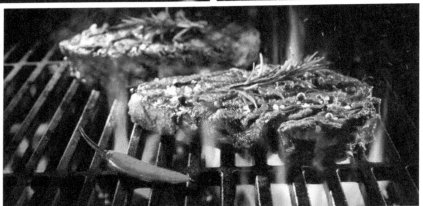

TRAEGER GRILL & SMOKER COOKBOOK

WOOD PELLET GRILL GUIDE WITH RECIPES&TIPS TO ENJOY
SMOKED FOOD. EARN PITMASTER STATUS AMONG YOUR
FRIENDS AND FAMILY!

OLIVER ROSS

TABLE OF CONTENTS

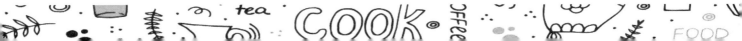

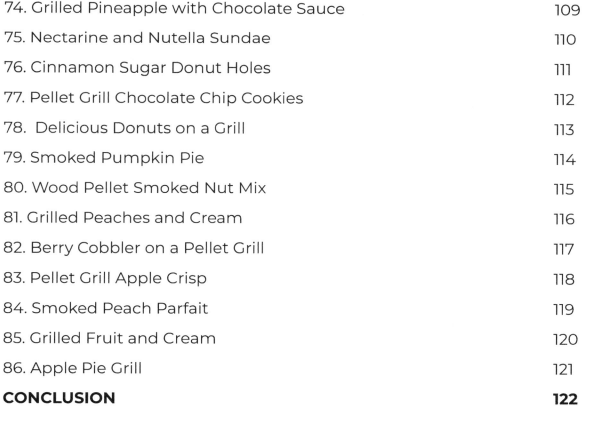

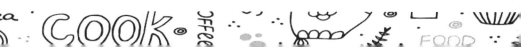

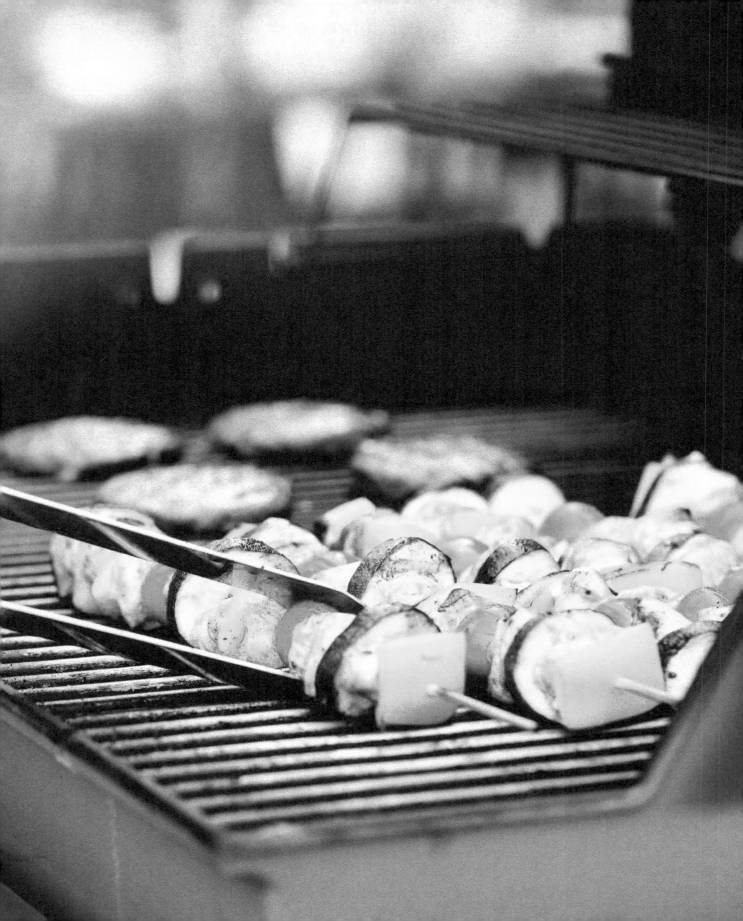

INTRODUCTION

Traeger wood pellets are currently all the rage and are the reason behind that delicious, moist, and tender smoked ribs in gatherings. These wood pellets appeal to pros and beginners alike by producing a classic barbecue right at your home. It all started in the 1980s when Joe Traeger started experimenting with pellet stoves, which have evolved into the famous Traeger wood pellet grill.

Traeger wood pellet grill uses wood pellets, which are twice the size of a pencil eraser, to grill smoke and bake foods. The Traeger heats the pellets that in turn, heat the cooking chamber, thus cooking food directly or indirectly. The wood pellets come in a wide range of flavors that are infused in food, taking their taste profile to the next level.

ESSENTIALS OF A TRAEGER WOOD PELLET GRILL

Wood Pellets

They are the main fuel in the Traeger, and you can choose the flavor of wood pellets you want to use, including hickory, cherry, apple, maple, mesquite, oak, among others.

Hopper

It's where the wood pellets are stored, awaiting combustion. You should always keep your hopper well loaded with enough wood pellets of your desired flavor.

Auger

This is a screw-like device that feeds the firepot with wood pellets.

Firepot

The wood pellets are ignited and burnt here to produce heat that cooks food. It's wise to empty the ashes in the firepot after cooking to maintain its efficiency.

Igniter Rod

It is located at the end of the auger and ignites the wood pellets in the firepot depending on if you want to fire or smoke.

Induction Fan

The induction fan turns on as soon as you turn on the grill. It ensures a constant flow of air resulting in conventional cooking.

Controller

The controller allows you to choose and regulate the desired temperature while cooking.

Drip Pan

It allows heat to pass through, prevents the fire from directly burning the food, and prevents the grease runoff from reaching the fire.

How Traeger Wood Pellet Grill Works

The wood pellets are poured into the hopper, where the auger feeds the pellets to the firepot. The ignition rod ignites the pellets that produce fire or rich hardwood smoke. An induction fan diffuses heat and smoke through the drip tray. The heats cook the food on the grill grates depending on the method you want to use: grilling, baking, smoking, among others.

The Traeger also has a controller that helps control the amount of heat you cook with as easy as in a conventional oven. Also, the grill thermostat determines the best time to add pellets in the firebox, thus maintaining constant heat. Not forgetting the Temperature display that uses a built-in thermal sensor to indicate the current cooking temperature.

Traeger Wood Pellet Grill vs. Charcoal and Wood Grills

People are always asking which is better: a pellet grill or a charcoal grill. While both can be used to smoke and grill food, their operation is totally different.

Let's discuss some differences between the two:

Flavor Impact

Wood pellet grill uses wood to cook, thus the taste of wood in the finished product. It can also cook under controlled low temperatures. Charcoal grill, on the other hand, gives food unmistakable charcoal flavor. The high temperatures also give the meat a good sear.

Cost

Traeger wood pellet grill is relatively expensive compared to most charcoal burners. This doesn't mean you can't get a charcoal grill that costs as much as a wood pellet, but you can get a charcoal grill at a very low price.

Operating Cost

Some wood pellet brands are more expensive than others. The expensive pellets tend not to jam up the auger, unlike the inexpensive pellets. You may also be required to repair or replace some Traeger parts if it breaks down outside the warranty period.

Charcoal briquettes are inexpensive with lump charcoal being more expensive. Many people prefer lump charcoal over briquettes.

Ease of Use

A Traeger wood pellet grill is very easy to use since you just need to feed the hopper with pellets and set the desired temperatures. In case you turn up the temperatures, it triggers an increase of pellets in the firebox, creating a hotter fire.

Charcoal grill, on the other hand, requires some expertise. Lighting up the charcoal may take 20-30 minutes, then reaching the desired temperature is a hustle. You will also be required to learn how to control airflow.

Temperature Control

Controlling the temperature in digital wood pellets is as easy as turning the dial and setting the temperature. In a charcoal grill, you control the temperatures by opening and closing the vents. The more air gets through the charcoal grill, the hotter it gets and the vice versa.

Run Time

Most wood pellets are designed to run more than 8 hours without adding the pellets. In case the pellets run low, there is no need to open the hopper lid to dump more pellets. Charcoal grills, on the other hand, can run up to 12 or more hours when smoking or cooking at low temperatures. It's also possible to burn all charcoal in a few hours.

CHAPTER 1. FUNDAMENTALS OF THE TRAEGER GRILL

With so many grills that are available in the market, the Traeger Grill is considered one of the best grills that you can ever invest in your outdoor kitchen. This innovative grill allows you to cook authentic grilled foods, yet you don't deviate from the tradition of cooking using wood pellets, so you don't get that distasteful aftertaste you get from cooking in a gas grill.

Made by an Oregon-based company, the Traeger Grill has been around for many decades. This type of smoker grill is known to cook food using all-nature wood pellets so that foods do not only smell and taste great but also healthy. But unlike traditional smokers, the Traeger Grill has been innovated to provide convenience even to grill and barbecue neophytes. It comes with a motor that turns the auger, thereby consistently feeding the burn pot so you can achieve even cooking.

THE ADVANTAGES OF TRAEGER GRILL

The Traeger Grill is not only limited to, well, grilling. It is an essential outdoor kitchen appliance as it allows you to also bake, roast, smoke, braise, and barbecue. But more than being a useful kitchen appliance, below are the advantages of getting your very own Traeger Grill:

- Better flavor: The Traeger Grill uses all-natural wood, so food comes out better-tasting compared to when you cook them in a gas or charcoal grill.

- No flare-ups: No flare-ups mean that food is cooked evenly on all sides. This is made possible by using indirect heat. And because there are no flare-ups, you can smoke, bake, and rose without some areas or sides of your food burning.

- Mechanical parts are well designed and protected: The mechanical parts of the Traeger Grill are protected, particularly from fats and drippings, so it does not get stuck over time.

- Exceptional temperature control: The Traeger Grill has exceptional temperature control. The thing is that all you need is to set up the heat, and the grill will maintain a consistent temperature even if the weather goes bad. Moreover, having a stable temperature control allows you to cook food better and tastier because of the burnt taste.

- Built-in Wi-Fi: All Traeger Grills have built-in Wi-Fi, so you can set them up even if you are not physically present in front of your grill. Moreover, the grill also alerts you once your food is ready. With this setting, you will be able to do other important things instead of slaving in front of your grill. Lastly, it also comes with an app that allows you to check many recipes from their website.

- Environmentally friendly: Perhaps the main selling point of the Traeger Grill is that it is environmentally friendly. Traeger Grill uses all-natural wood pellets, so your grill does not produce harmful chemicals when you are using it... only smoky goodness.

The thing is that the Traeger Grill is more than just your average grill. It is one of the best there is, and you will definitely get your money's worth with this grill.

CONTROL PANEL

While the Traeger Grill is designed to be innovative, operating it is no rocket science. In fact, the standard digital controller or control panel of the Traeger grill is extremely easy to understand, even for someone who is a novice in the kitchen.

- Temperature Panel: The temperature panel indicates the temperature that you want to maintain while cooking your food. Temperature is displayed in Fahrenheit.

- Temperature Control Knob: The temperature knob allows you to increase or decrease the temperature in increments of 25 degrees. The temperature range is from 180°F to 375°F. The temperature control knob also comes with options such as Smoke, High Temperature, and Shut Down Cycle.

- Timer: The latest models of Traeger Grills also comes with a timer so that your food cooks at the proper moment. This option is also especially important as you do not need to be in front of your grill to turn it off.

- Menu: More advanced Traeger Grills come with a menu setting that allows you to control your grill settings. You can also update the firmware version of your grill so that you can optimize its Wi-Fi connectivity.

WHAT TO DO BEFORE START

Grill Placement

Grills can cause fires, so setting up your unit in the proper location can go a long way in protecting your home and family. So, remember to place the grill:

- A good distance from deck railings, awnings, and similar structures as well as trees with overhanging branches and piles of dry grass or leaves.

- Away from paint and aerosol cans, gasoline, vehicles, and machines that contain gasoline.

Lid Up or Lid Down

There are pros and cons to keeping the lid up or down while you grill, and the best choice depends in part on the food you're cooking.

Keeping the grill open, with the lid up, is like cooking food directly over a camp fire. Direct heat equals higher temperatures, so food tends to cook faster. But because of the lack of surrounding heat, you need to turn food often to make sure all sides are cooked evenly and thoroughly.

How to Setup Your Grill

The prep portion is all the work you do before you bring your food to the grill. The number one priority in the preparation cycle is advance planning. Give yourself plenty of time to read the recipe and explore the steps or procedures you might have questions about. Recipes may require cooling overnight or hours after preparation to allow rubs, spices, pickles, and marinades to work their magic. Before you start preparing, collect all the necessary ingredients and cooking equipment. If you do not use fresh meat, poultry, or seafood, make sure the proteins are thawed in the refrigerator before release. Above all, ensure proper sanitation.

There will come a time when cycles of preparation and orientation can occur simultaneously. Depending on the preheating time of your pellet grill, as with a traditional closed oven, you can choose to preheat while preparation is complete.

How to Fire Up Your Grill and Smoker

For Preferred Wood Pellet or charcoal smoker, first, light up half of the charcoals and wait until their flame goes down. Then add remaining charcoal and Preferred Wood Pellet chips if using. Wait, they are lighted and giving heat completely, then push charcoal aside and place the meat on the other side of the grilling grate. This is done to make sure that meat is indirectly smoked over low heat. Continue adding charcoal and/or soaked Preferred Wood Pellet chips into the smoker.

Tips

- Cooking Times: Always determine the cooking time based on the reading of the internal food temperature and the cooking time I have given you.

- Pre-Heating: The time your wood pellet is heated can vary from manufacturer to startup procedure. The main thing is to do some tests and know your grill.

- Clean Food: Always keep the food in the refrigerator to keep it safe and prevent disease; soak it in cold water, replacing the water every 30 minutes, keeping the food submerged; or use the microwave defrost setting. Do not defrost frozen food on your work surface.

- Internal Temperature: Always cook at internal temperatures using an instant-read digital thermometer.

- Voltage: Most recipes require you to put protein in an aluminum tent before slicing or serving. Carp is an easy technique. Fold in the middle of the sheet of aluminum foil, roll in a tent, and place without pressure on the food.

- Skin Protection: Wear nitrile gloves without food when handling raw meat and hot peppers like jalapeños.

- Sole Treatment: Solely for curing, used in some tiles and sports recipes, it has salt and nitrite and should never be used for seasonal table food or cooking.

- Note on Smoke: The higher the temperature, the less smoker smokes on the grill with pellets. This unit will not produce visible strength above 300°F. Therefore, use granules of your choice when a higher temperature is reached because the granule granules will not affect the taste.

CHAPTER 2. TIPS FOR GRILLING SUCCESS

PELLET STORAGE

You have to be vigilant in storing your pellets, especially if you live in a humid climate. Damp or wet pellets will not lead to the best grilling experience—you won't be able to get a fire going. What's worse, damp or wet pellets will damage the auger since it won't be able to rotate and will burn out the motor.

TEMPERATURE READINGS

After using your grill a few times, you may notice that the temperature starts to fluctuate quite a bit. This is because of grease and soot build-up on the temperature probe used to regulate the temperature. An effortless way to stop this from happening is to clean the probe and cover it with foil. Consequently, cooking temperature readings will be more accurate.

COVER YOUR GRILL

You may think a grill cover isn't necessary, but believe me, it's crucial. Your Traeger grill is an appliance and one with electronics inside to boot! If you want to ensure your pellet smoker's durability, protect it from the elements. If you can, move your grill under a rooftop after having a barbeque and use a grill cover. You don't want your pellet smoker to stop working suddenly due to water damage.

CLEAN YOUR GRILL

A lot of people fail at keeping their grill clean. This step is crucial to guard against overfilling the fire pot and protect against flare-ups. Not to mention that your grill will look brand-new for longer if you care for it in this simple way. I recommend cleaning your Traeger grill after cooking something for an extended period or after you're done using it for the weekend. If you love cooking greasier foods, you'll have to clean your grill more often. Here are the steps you should follow:

1. Use an all-natural degreaser/cleaner to spray the grill grate and the inside of the chimney.

2. Remove and clean the sides of the grill grates.

3. Throw away the old foil and drip tray liners.

4. Remove the drip tray and heat baffle.

5. Use a vacuum inside the grill and fire pot to remove any food particles.

6. Clean the inside of the chimney.

7. Again use an all-natural degreaser/cleaner to spray the inside and outside of the grill. Wait a few minutes before wiping clean.

8. Put all components back in their place, including the heat baffle, drip tray, and foil liners. You're all set for your next barbeque!

Tip: Avoid using wire brushes as it will scratch your Traeger grill. Heavy-duty paper towels or a cleaning cloth will work nicely.

BE ADVENTUROUS

This is vital to your grilling success—you won't enjoy your Traeger grill for long if you have to make the same recipes over and over. What's more, you own a 6-in-1 appliance, and you can't let that versatility go unused. In the beginning, as you get used to a pellet grill, you may end up cooking simple meals, but once you feel confident in your grilling abilities, try new things! Don't limit yourself to cooking only traditional barbeque foods—what about making a smoky bean stew in your Traeger grill? Don't worry; later on in this cookbook, you'll see recipes that will spark your adventurous side.

These aren't the only elements that will contribute to your grilling success, but they cover some of the rookie mistakes many people, myself included, make. It put a real downer on my grilling plans!

COOKING TIME AND TEMPERATURES

MEAT	COOKING TEMPERATURE	COOKING TIME
BEEF SHORT RIBS	225 °F TO 250 °F	4 TO 6 HOURS
BEEF TENDERLOIN (MEDIUM RARE)	225 °F TO 250 °F	2.5 TO 3 HOURS
BEEF TRI-TIP (MEDIUM)	225 °F TO 250 °F	3 TO 3.5 HOURS
BELLY BACON	LESS THAN 100 °F	6 HOURS
BONELESS PRIME RIB	225 °F TO 250 °F	12 MINUTES/LB.
BRISKET (PULLED) 8-12 LBS.	225 °F TO 250 °F	1.5 HOURS/LB.
BUTT BACON	LESS THAN 100 °F	6 HOURS
CHICKEN (WHOLE) 2.5-3 LBS.	275 °F TO 350 °F	2 TO 2.5 HOURS
CHICKEN (QUARTERS)	275 °F TO 350 °F	1 TO 2 HOURS
CHICKEN (THIGHS)	275 °F TO 350 °F	1.5 HOURS

CHICKEN (WINGS)	275 °F TO 350 °F	1.25 HOURS
CHUCK ROAST (MEDIUM)	225 °F TO 250 °F	1.25 HOURS
FILET MIGNON	COLD SMOKE THEN 350 °F	UNTIL DONE
FISH (FILLETS)	225 °F TO 240 °F	1.5 TO 2 HOURS
HAM (BONE IN)	225 °F TO 250 °F	1.5 HOURS/LB.
PORK CHOPS	225 °F TO 250 °F	1.5 HOURS/LB.
PORK SHOULDER (PULLED) 6-10 LBS.	225 °F TO 250 °F	8 TO 12 HOURS
PRIME RIB	225 °F TO 250 °F	15 MIN/LB.
RUMP ROAST	225 °F TO 250 °F	30 MIN/LB.
SMOKED HAMBURGERS	225 °F TO 250 °F	30 TO 40 MIN

CARING FOR YOUR TRAEGER GRILL

You've invested in your pellet smoker, and I'm sure you want to know the best way to care for it and make sure it lasts you through the years. I talked about the importance of regularly cleaning your grill and what steps to follow, resulting in a more superficial clean. This is more than adequate for the short-term. However, you will have to give your Traeger grill a deep clean every few months. Think of it as spring cleaning your pellet smoker.

EVERY SIX MONTHS: CLEAN THE SMOKE STACK

1. Unscrew the chimney cap after you're hundred percent sure the grill is cold.

2. Use a non-metallic tool to rub any build-up from both the vertical and horizontal segments of the smokestack.

3. Use a paper towel or cloth to remove any remaining residue.

4. You can use a biodegradable degreaser to clean the chimney cap if needed.

EVERY THREE TO SIX MONTHS: CLEAN THE GREASE DRIP

1. Wait for your grill to cool and remove the grease bucket.

2. Use a wooden or silicone tool to scrape any grease from the drain located at the bottom of the drip tray. Also, clean the tube leading to the grease bucket.

3. Use disposable rags or paper towels to remove any residue.

4. Scrape grease from the grease bucket with a non-metallic tool. Then wipe off any residual fat.

Every Three Months: Clean Outside

1. Make sure the grill is cold and disconnect the power cord.

2. Use a cleaning cloth or disposable rag and warm soapy water to clean any visible grease from the outside. Do not use any abrasive cleaners.

3. Apply a high-quality car wax to the outside surfaces.

Answering Your Questions

There may be some technical issues with any appliances, primarily since your Traeger Grill and Smoker work with electricity. Here are some of the most frequently asked questions when it comes to general use and troubleshooting.

My Grill Isn't Lighting; What Am I Doing Wrong?

This can happen due to the hotrod not heating up, the induction fan not working, or the auger isn't feeding the fire pot with pellets. Use a process of elimination to find the source of the problem.

My Traeger Grill and Smoker Doesn't Want to Power On. Why?

It's usually due to some or other electrical issues. It can be a bad power outlet, a bad extension cord, a blown fuse on the controller, or the GFCI tripped.

My Auger Isn't Moving

If you used damp pellets, it might have caused your auger to jam. If that's not the case, the shear pin that holds the motor to the auger may be broken. You can also check if the auger motor is in working order and make sure that it is getting power from the controller.

The Induction Fan Isn't Running

If you haven't used your pellet smoker in a while, the grease on the fan base may have seized—give it a spin to loosen it. In addition, check if there is power from the controller to the orange wires. Lastly, make sure there isn't an obstruction keeping your fan from turning.

My Grill Is Running Hot on Smoke. Why is This?

The outside weather will play a role in the smoke temperature since it will have to compensate for hotter or colder conditions. It might also be a case of you closing the lid too soon after the grill was started. It is best to leave the top open for at least 10 minutes to give the startup fuel time to burn off.

Can I Use Firebricks in My Pellet Grill?

That is not recommended.

How Long Can I Leave My Traeger Grill Unattended?

It would be best if you kept the hopper at least half full at all times. So, if you know you're grilling at a high temperature, you will have to check on the level of pellets in the hopper regularly. You can expect to use 3 lbs. per hour when cooking at higher temperatures.

Do I Always Have to Use Pellets?

Since pellets are the heat source of your smoker, you won't be able to use your Traeger grill without it.

That should answer some questions you may face at some point in time when using your Traeger Grill and Smoker! I hope, after reading this chapter, you feel confident enough to use your pellet grill. If you're still not sure, the recipes ahead will convince you to grab your wood pellets, tongs and get cooking!

Remember, there's no reason why you shouldn't get creative; use these recipes as a guide, and soon you'll be coming up with your very own barbeque masterpieces. Just imagine how popular you'll be at the next neighborhood BBQ!

CHAPTER 3. FISH AND SEAFOOD RECIPES

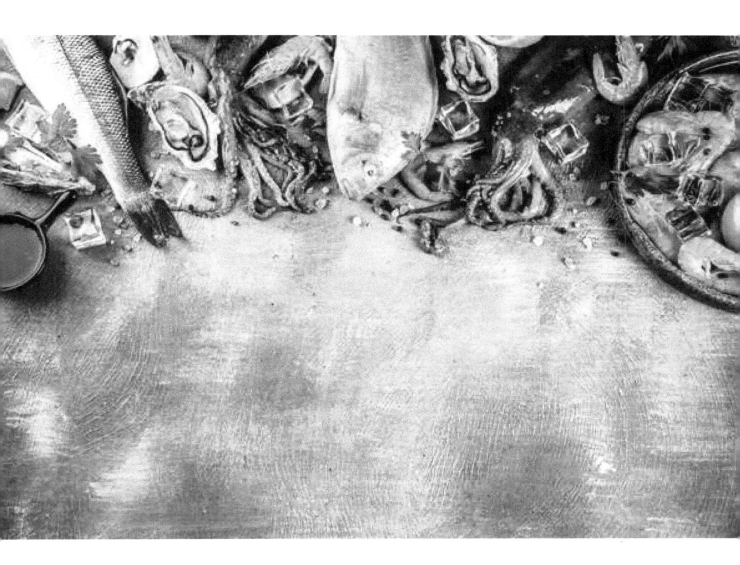

1. BLACKENED CATFISH

INGREDIENTS

Spice blend:

- 1 teaspoon granulated garlic
- 1/4 teaspoon cayenne pepper
- 1/2 cup Cajun seasoning
- 1 teaspoon ground thyme
- 1 teaspoon ground oregano
- 1 teaspoon onion powder
- 1 tablespoon smoked paprika
- 1 teaspoon pepper.

Fish:

- 4 catfish fillets
- Salt to taste
- 1/2 cup butter.

DIRECTIONS

1. In a bowl, combine all the ingredients for the spice blend.
2. Sprinkle both sides of the fish with the salt and spice blend.
3. Set your wood pellet grill to 450 degrees F.
4. Heat your cast iron pan and add the butter. Add the fillets to the pan.
5. Cook for 5 minutes per side.
6. Serving Suggestion: Garnish with lemon wedges.
7. Tip: Smoke the catfish for 20 minutes before seasoning.

Nutritions: Calories: 181.5 Fat: 10.5g Cholesterol: 65.8mg Carbohydrates: 2.9g Fiber: 1.8g Sugars: 0.4g Protein: 19.2g.

2. BACON-WRAPPED SCALLOPS

INGREDIENTS

- 12 scallops
- 12 bacon slices
- 3 tablespoons lemon juice
- Pepper to taste.

DIRECTIONS

1. Turn on your wood pellet grill.
2. Set it to smoke.
3. Let it burn for 5 minutes while the lid is open.
4. Set it to 400 degrees F.
5. Wrap the scallops with bacon.
6. Secure with a toothpick.
7. Drizzle with the lemon juice and season with pepper.
8. Add the scallops to a baking tray.
9. Place the tray on the grill.
10. Grill for 20 minutes.
11. Serving Suggestion: Serve with sweet chili sauce.

Nutritions: Calories: 180.3 Fat: 8g Cholesterol: 590.2mg Carbohydrates: 3g Fiber: 0g Sugars: 0g Protein: 22g.

3. CAJUN SEASONED SHRIMP

INGREDIENTS

- 20 pieces of jumbo shrimp
- 1/2 teaspoon of cajun seasoning
- 1 tablespoon of canola oil
- 1 teaspoon of magic shrimp seasoning.

DIRECTIONS

1. Take a large bowl and add canola oil, shrimp, and seasonings.
2. Mix well for fine coating.
3. Now put the shrimp on skewers.
4. Put the grill grate inside the grill and set a timer to 8 minutes at high for preheating.
5. Once the grill is preheated, open the unit and place the shrimp skewers inside.
6. Cook the shrimp for 2 minutes.
7. Open the unit to flip the shrimp and cook for another 2 minutes at medium.
8. Own done, serve.

Nutritions: Calories: 382 Total Fat: 7.4g Saturated Fat: 0g Cholesterol: 350mg Sodium: 2208mg Tota Carbohydrates: 23.9g Dietary Fiber: 2.6g Total Sugars: 2.6g Protein: 50.2g.

4. JUICY SMOKED SALMON

INGREDIENTS

- ½ cup of sugar
- 2 tablespoon salt
- 2 tablespoons crushed red pepper flakes
- ½ cup fresh mint leaves, chopped
- ¼ cup brandy
- 1 (4 pounds) salmon, bones removed
- 2 cups alder wood pellets, soaked in water.

DIRECTIONS

1. Take a medium-sized bowl and add brown sugar, crushed red pepper flakes, mint leaves, salt, and brandy until a paste forms.
2. Rub the paste all over your salmon and wrap the salmon with a plastic wrap.
3. Allow them to chill overnight.
4. Preheat your smoker to 220 degrees Fahrenheit and add wood Pellets.
5. Transfer the salmon to the smoker rack and cook smoke for 45 minutes.
6. Once the salmon has turned red-brown and the flesh flakes off easily, take it out and serve!

Nutritions: Calories: 370 Fats: 28g Carbs: 1g Fiber: 0g.

5. PEPPERCORN TUNA STEAKS

INGREDIENTS

- ¼ cup of salt
- 2 pounds yellowfin tuna
- ¼ cup Dijon mustard
- Freshly ground black pepper
- 2 tablespoons peppercorn.

DIRECTIONS

1. Take a large-sized container and dissolve salt in warm water (enough water to cover fish).
2. Transfer tuna to the brine and cover, refrigerate for 8 hours.
3. Preheat your smoker to 250 degrees Fahrenheit with your preferred wood.
4. Remove tuna from bring and pat it dry.
5. Transfer to grill pan and spread Dijon mustard all over.
6. Season with pepper and sprinkle peppercorn on top.
7. Transfer tuna to smoker and smoker for 1 hour.
8. Enjoy!

Nutritions: Calories: 707 Fats: 57g Carbs: 10g Fiber: 2g.

6. STUFFED SHRIMP TILAPIA

INGREDIENTS

- 5 ounces fresh, farmed tilapia fillets
- 2 tablespoons extra virgin olive oil
- 1 and ½ teaspoons smoked paprika
- 1 and ½ teaspoons Old Bay seasoning
- Shrimp stuffing
- 1 pound shrimp, cooked and deveined
- 1 tablespoon salted butter
- 1 cup red onion, diced
- 1 cup Italian bread crumbs
- ½ cup mayonnaise
- 1 large egg, beaten
- 2 teaspoons fresh parsley, chopped
- 1 and ½ teaspoons salt and pepper.

DIRECTIONS

1. Take a food processor and add shrimp, chop them up.
2. Take a skillet and place it over medium-high heat, add butter and allow it to melt.
3. Sauté the onions for 3 minutes.
4. Add chopped shrimp with cooled Sautéed onion alongside remaining ingredients listed under stuffing ingredients and transfer to a bowl.
5. Cover the mixture and allow it to refrigerate for 60 minutes.
6. Rub both sides of the fillet with olive oil.
7. Spoon 1/3 cup of the stuffing to the fillet.
8. Flatten out the stuffing onto the bottom half of the fillet and fold the Tilapia in half.
9. Secure with 2 toothpicks.
10. Dust each fillet with smoked paprika and Old Bay seasoning.
11. Preheat your smoker to 400 degrees Fahrenheit.
12. Add your preferred wood Pellets and transfer the fillets to a non-stick grill tray.
13. Transfer to your smoker and smoker for 30-45 minutes until the internal temperature reaches 145 degrees Fahrenheit.
14. Allow the fish to rest for 5 minutes and enjoy!

Nutritions: Calories: 620 Fats: 50g Carbs: 6g Fiber: 1g.

7. TOGARASHI SMOKED SALMON

INGREDIENTS

- 2 large Salmon filet
- Togarashi for seasoning
- For Brine:
- 1 cup brown sugar
- 4 cups water
- ⅓ cup kosher salt.

DIRECTIONS

1. Remove all the thorns from the fish filet.
2. Mix all the brine ingredients until the brown sugar is dissolved completely.
3. Put the mix in a big bowl and add the filet to it.
4. Leave the bowl to refrigerate for 16 hours.
5. After 16 hours, remove the salmon from this mix. Wash and dry it.
6. Place the salmon in the refrigerator for another 2-4 hours. (This step is important. DO NOT SKIP IT.)
7. Season your salmon filet with Togarashi.
8. Start the wood pellet grill with the 'smoke' option and place the salmon on it.
9. Smoke for 4 hours.
10. Make sure the temperature does not go above 180 degrees or below 130 degrees.
11. Remove from the grill and serve it warm with a side dish of your choice.

Nutritions: Carbohydrates: 19g Protein: 10g Fat: 6g Sodium: 3772mg Cholesterol: 29mg.

8. BBQ OYSTERS

INGREDIENTS

- 12 shucked oysters
- 1 lb. unsalted butter
- 1 bunch chopped green onions
- 1 tbsp. honey Hog BBQ Rub or Meat Church "The Gospel"
- ½ bunch minced green onions
- ½ cup seasoned breadcrumbs
- 2 cloves of minced garlic
- 8 oz. shredded pepper jack cheese
- Traeger Heat and Sweet BBQ sauce.

DIRECTIONS

1. Preheat the pellet grill for about 10-15 minutes with the lid closed.
2. To make the compound butter, wait for the butter to soften. Then combine the butter, onions, BBQ rub, and garlic thoroughly.
3. Lay the butter evenly on plastic wrap or parchment paper. Roll it up in a log shape and tie the ends with butcher's twine. Place these in the freezer to solidify for an hour. This butter can be used on any kind of grilled meat to enhance its flavor. Any other high-quality butter can also replace this compound butter.
4. Shuck the oysters, keeping the juice in the shell.
5. Sprinkle all the oysters with breadcrumbs and place them directly on the grill. Allow them to cook for 5 minutes. You will know they are cooked when the oysters begin to curl slightly at the edges.
6. Once they are cooked, put a spoonful of the compound butter on the oysters. Once the butter melts, you can add a little bit of pepper jack cheese to add more flavor to them.
7. The oysters must not be on the grill for longer than 6 minutes, or you risk overcooking them. Put a generous squirt of the BBQ sauce on all the oysters. Also, add a few chopped onions.
8. Allow them to cool for a few minutes and enjoy the taste of the sea!

Nutritions: Carbohydrates: 2.5g Protein: 4.7g Fat: 1.1g Sodium: 53mg Cholesterol: 25mg.

CHAPTER 4. POULTRY RECIPES

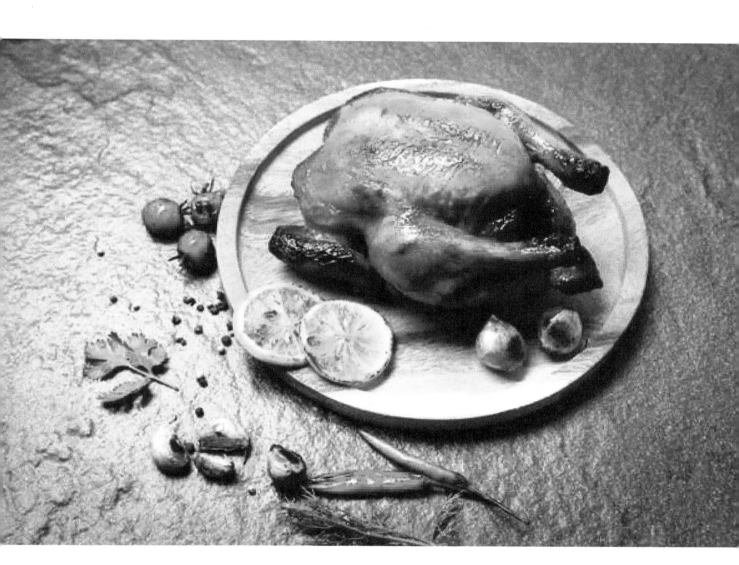

9. SWEET SRIRACHA BBQ CHICKEN

INGREDIENTS

- 1 cup sriracha
- ½ cup butter
- ½ cup molasses
- ½ cup ketchup
- ¼ cup firmly packed brown sugar
- 1 teaspoon salt
- 1 teaspoon fresh ground black pepper
- 1 whole chicken, cut into pieces
- ½ teaspoon fresh parsley leaves, chopped.

DIRECTIONS

1. Preheat your smoker to 250 degrees Fahrenheit using cherry wood.
2. Take a medium saucepan and place it over low heat, stir in butter, sriracha, ketchup, molasses, brown sugar, mustard, pepper, and salt and keep stirring until the sugar and salt dissolves.
3. Divide the sauce into two portions.
4. Brush the chicken half with the sauce and reserve the remaining for serving.
5. Make sure to keep the sauce for serving on the side and keep the other portion for basting.
6. Transfer chicken to your smoker rack and smoke for about 1 and a ½ to 2 hours until the internal temperature reaches 165 degrees Fahrenheit.
7. Sprinkle chicken with parsley and serve with reserved BBQ sauce.
8. Enjoy!

Nutritions: Calories: 148 Fats: 0.6g Carbs: 10g Fiber: 1g.

10. SMOKED CHICKEN DRUMSTICKS

INGREDIENTS

- 10 chicken drumsticks
- 2 tsp. garlic powder
- 1 tsp. salt
- 1 tsp. onion powder
- 1/2 tsp. ground black pepper
- ½ tsp. cayenne pepper
- 1 tsp. brown sugar
- 1/3 cup hot sauce
- 1 tsp. paprika
- ½ tsp. thyme.

DIRECTIONS

1. In a large mixing bowl, combine the garlic powder, sugar, hot sauce, paprika, thyme, cayenne, salt, and ground pepper. Add the drumsticks and toss to combine.
2. Cover the bowl and refrigerate for 1 hour.
3. Remove the drumsticks from the marinade and let them sit for about 1 hour until they are at room temperature.
4. Arrange the drumsticks into a rack.
5. Start your pellet grill on smoke, leaving the lid open for 5 minutes for the fire to start.
6. Close the lid and preheat grill to 250°F, using hickory or apple hardwood pellets.
7. Place the rack on the grill and smoke drumsticks for 2 hours, 30 minutes, or until the drumsticks' internal temperature reaches 180°F.
8. Remove drumsticks from heat and let them rest for a few minutes.
9. Serve.

Nutritions: Calories: 167 Total Fat: 5.4g Saturated Fat: 1.4g Cholesterol: 81mg Sodium: 946mg Total Carbohydrates: 2.6g Dietary Fiber: 0.5g Total Sugars: 1.3g Protein: 25.7g.

11. CHICKEN CORDON BLEU

INGREDIENTS

- 6 boneless skinless chicken breasts
- 6 slices of ham
- 12 slices Swiss cheese
- 1 cup panko breadcrumbs
- ½ cup all-purpose flour
- 1 tsp. ground black pepper or to taste
- 1 tsp. salt or to taste
- 4 tbsp. grated parmesan cheese
- 2 tbsp. melted butter
- ½ tsp. garlic powder
- ½ tsp. thyme
- ¼ tsp. parsley.

DIRECTIONS

1. Butterfly the chicken breast with a pairing knife. Place the chicken breast in between 2 plastic wraps and pound with a mallet until the chicken breasts are ¼ inch thick.
2. Place a plastic wrap on a flat surface. Place one fat chicken breast on it.
3. Place one slice of Swiss cheese on the chicken. Place one slice of ham over the cheese and place another cheese slice over the ham.
4. Roll the chicken breast tightly. Fold both ends of the roll tightly. Pin both ends of the rolled chicken breast with a toothpick.
5. Repeat step 3 and 4 for the remaining chicken breasts
6. In a mixing bowl, combine the all-purpose flour, ½ tsp. salt, and ½ tsp. pepper. Set aside.
7. In another mixing bowl, combine breadcrumbs, parmesan, butter, garlic, thyme, parsley, ½ tsp. salt, and ½ tsp. pepper. Set aside.
8. Break the eggs into another mixing bowl and whisk. Set aside.
9. Grease a baking sheet.
10. Bake one chicken breast roll. Dip into the flour mixture, brush with eggs and dip into breadcrumb mixture. The chicken breast should be coated.
11. Place it on the baking sheet.
12. Repeat steps 9 and 10 for the remaining breast rolls.
13. Preheat your grill to 375°F with the lid closed for 15 minutes.
14. Place the baking sheet on the grill and cook for about 40 minutes, or until the chicken is golden brown.
15. Remove the baking sheet from the grill and let the chicken rest for a few minutes.
16. Slice cordon bleu and serve.

Nutritions: Calories: 560 Total Fat: 27.4g Saturated Fat: 15.9g Cholesterol: 156mg Sodium: 1158mg Total Carbohydrates: 23.2g Dietary Fiber: 1.1g Total Sugars: 1.2g Protein: 54.3g.

12. WOOD PELLET GRILLED CHICKEN KABOBS

INGREDIENTS

- 1/2 cup olive oil
- 2 tbsp. white vinegar
- 1 tbsp. lemon juice
- 1-1/2 tbsp. salt
- 1/2 tbsp. pepper, coarsely ground
- 2 tbsp. chives, freshly chopped
- 1-1/2 tbsp. thyme, freshly chopped
- 2 tbsp. Italian parsley freshly chopped
- 1tbsp. garlic, minced
- Kabobs
- 1 each orange, red, and yellow pepper
- 1-1/2 pounds chicken breast, boneless and skinless
- 12 mini mushrooms.

DIRECTIONS

1. In a mixing bowl, add all the marinade ingredients and mix well. Toss the chicken and mushrooms in the marinade, then refrigerate for 30 minutes.
2. Meanwhile, soak the skewers in hot water. Remove the chicken from the fridge and start assembling the kabobs.
3. Preheat your wood pellet to 450°F.
4. Grill the kabobs in the wood pellet for 6 minutes, flip them, and grill for 6 more minutes.
5. Remove from the grill and let rest. Heat up the naan bread on the grill for 2 minutes.
6. Serve and enjoy.

Nutritions: Calories: 165 Fat: 13g Carbohydrates: 1g Protein: 33g Fiber: 0g.

13. WOOD PELLET GRILLED CHICKEN

INGREDIENTS

- 5 pounds whole chicken
- 1/2 cup oil
- Chicken rub.

DIRECTIONS

1. Preheat your wood pellet on smoke with the lid open for 5 minutes. Close the lid, increase the temperature to 450°F and preheat for 15 more minutes.
2. Tie the chicken legs together with the baker's twine, then rub the chicken with oil and coat with chicken rub.
3. Place the chicken on the grill with the breast side up.
4. Grill the chicken for 70 minutes without opening it or until the internal temperature reaches 165°F.
5. Once the chicken is out of the grill, let it cool down for 15 minutes
6. Enjoy.

Nutritions: Calories: 935 Fat: 53g Carbohydrates: 0g Protein: 107g Fiber: 0g.

14. WOOD PELLET CHICKEN BREASTS

INGREDIENTS

- 3 chicken breasts
- 1 tbsp. avocado oil
- 1/4 tbsp. garlic powder
- 1/4 tbsp. onion powder
- 3/4 tbsp. salt
- 1/4 tbsp. pepper.

DIRECTIONS

1. Preheat your pellet to 375°F.
2. Half the chicken breasts lengthwise, then coat with avocado oil.
3. With the spices, drizzle it on all sides to season
4. Drizzle spices to season the chicken. Put the chicken on top of the grill and begin to cook until its internal temperature approaches 165 degrees Fahrenheit. Put the chicken on top of the grill and begin to cook until it rises to a temperature of 165 degrees Fahrenheit
5. Serve and enjoy.

Nutritions: Calories: 120 Fat: 4g Carbohydrates: 0g Protein: 19g Fiber: 0g.

15. WOOD PELLET SMOKED SPATCHCOCK TURKEY

INGREDIENTS

- 1 whole turkey
- 1/2 cup oil
- 1/4 cup chicken rub
- 1 tbsp. onion powder
- 1 tbsp. garlic powder
- 1 tbsp. rubbed sage.

DIRECTIONS

1. Preheat your wood pellet grill to high.
2. Meanwhile, place the turkey on a platter with the breast side down, then cut on either side of the backbone to remove the spine.
3. Flip the turkey and season on both sides, then place it on the preheated grill or on a pan if you want to catch the drippings. Grill on high for 30 minutes, reduce the temperature to 325°F, and grill for 45 more minutes or until the internal temperature reaches 165°F. Remove from the grill and let rest for 20 minutes before slicing and serving. Enjoy.

Nutritions: Calories: 156 Fat: 16g Carbohydrates: 1g Protein: 2g Fiber: 0g.

16. WOOD PELLET SMOKED CORNISH HENS

INGREDIENTS

- 6 Cornish hens
- 3 tbsp. avocado oil
- 6 tbsp. rub of choice.

DIRECTIONS

1. Fire up the wood pellet and preheat it to 275°F.
2. Rub the hens with oil, then coat generously with rub. Place the hens on the grill with the chest breast side down.
3. Smoke for 30 minutes. Flip the hens and increase the grill temperature to 400°F. Cook until the internal temperature reaches 165°F.
4. Remove from the grill and let rest for 10 minutes before serving. Enjoy.

Nutritions: Calories: 696 Fat: 50g Carbohydrates: 1g Protein: 57g Fiber: 0g.

17. SMOKED AND FRIED CHICKEN WINGS

INGREDIENTS

- 3 pounds chicken wings
- 1 tbsp. Goya adobo all-purpose seasoning
- Sauce of your choice.

DIRECTIONS

1. Fire up your wood pellet grill and set it to smoke.
2. Meanwhile, coat the chicken wings with all-purpose adobo seasoning. Place the chicken on the grill and smoke for 2 hours.
3. Remove the wings from the grill.
4. Preheat oil to 375°F in a frying pan. Drop the wings in batches and let fry for 5 minutes or until the skin is crispy.
5. Drain the oil and proceed with drizzling the preferred sauce.
6. Drain oil and drizzle preferred sauce.
7. Enjoy.

Nutritions: Calories: 755 Fat: 55g Carbohydrates: 24g Protein: 39g Fiber: 1g.

18. WOOD PELLET GRILLED BUFFALO CHICKEN LEG

INGREDIENTS

- 12 chicken legs
- 1/2 tbsp. salt
- 1 tbsp. buffalo seasoning
- 1 cup buffalo sauce.

DIRECTIONS

1. Preheat your wood pellet grill to 325°F.
2. Toss the legs in salt and buffalo seasoning, then place them on the preheated grill.
3. Grill for 40 minutes, ensuring you turn them twice through the cooking.
4. Brush the legs with buffalo sauce and cook for an additional 10 minutes or until the internal temperature reaches 165°F.
5. Remove the legs from the grill, brush with more sauce, and serve when hot.

Nutritions: Calories: 956 Fat: 47g Carbohydrates: 1g Protein: 124g Fiber: 0g.

19. WOOD PELLET CHILE LIME CHICKEN

INGREDIENTS

- 1 chicken breast
- 1 tbsp. oil
- 1 tbsp. chile-lime seasoning.

DIRECTIONS

1. Preheat your wood pellet to 400°F.
2. Brush the chicken breast with oil on all sides.
3. Sprinkle with seasoning and salt to taste.
4. Grill for 7 minutes per side or until the internal temperature reaches 165°F.
5. Serve when hot or cold and enjoy.

Nutritions: Calories: 131 Fat: 5g Carbohydrates: 4g Protein: 19g Fiber: 1g.

20. WOOD PELLET SHEET PAN CHICKEN FAJITAS

INGREDIENTS

- 2 tbsp. oil
- 2 tbsp. chile margarita seasoning
- 1 tbsp. salt
- 1/2 tbsp. onion powder
- 1/2 tbsp. garlic, granulated
- 2-pound chicken breast, thinly sliced
- 1 red bell pepper, seeded and sliced
- 1 orange bell pepper
- 1 onion, sliced.

DIRECTIONS

1. Preheat the wood pellet to 450°F. Meanwhile, mix oil and seasoning, then toss the chicken and the peppers. Line a sheet pan with foil, then place it in the preheated grill. Let it heat for 10 minutes with the grill's lid closed. Open the grill and place the chicken with the veggies on the pan in a single layer. Cook for 10 minutes or until the chicken is cooked and no longer pink. Remove from grill and serve with tortilla or your favorite fixings.

Nutritions: Calories: 211 Fat: 6g Carbohydrates: 5g Protein: 29g Fiber: 1g.

21. SMOKED WHOLE DUCK

INGREDIENTS

- 5 pounds whole duck (trimmed of any excess fat)
- 1 small onion (quartered)
- 1 apple (wedged)
- 1 orange (quartered)
- 1 tbsp. freshly chopped parsley
- 1 tbsp. freshly chopped sage
- ½ tsp. onion powder
- 2 tsp. smoked paprika
- 1 tsp. dried Italian seasoning
- 1 tbsp. dried Greek seasoning
- 1 tsp. pepper or to taste
- 1 tsp. sea salt or to taste.

DIRECTIONS

1. Remove giblets and rinse duck, inside and pour, under cold running water.
2. Pat dry with paper towels.
3. Use the tip of a sharp knife to cut the duck skin all over. Be careful not to cut through the meat. Tie the duck legs together with butcher's string.
4. To make a rub, combine the onion powder, pepper, salt, Italian seasoning, Greek seasoning, and paprika in a mixing bowl.
5. Insert the orange, onion, and apple into the duck cavity. Stuff the duck with freshly chopped parsley and sage.
6. Season all sides of the duck generously with rub mixture.
7. Start your pellet grill on smoke mode, leaving the lip open or until the fire starts.
8. Close the lid and preheat the grill to 325°F for 10 minutes.
9. Place the duck on the grill grate.
10. Roast for 2 to 21/2 hours, or until the duck skin is brown and the internal temperature of the thigh reaches 160°F.
11. Remove the duck from heat and let it rest for a few minutes.
12. Cut into sizes and serve.

Nutritions: Calories: 809 Total Fat: 42.9g Saturated Fat: 15.8g Cholesterol: 337mg Sodium: 638mg Total Carbohydrates: 11.7g Dietary Fiber: 2.4g Total Sugars: 7.5g Protein: 89.6g.

22. CHICKEN FAJITAS ON A WOOD PELLET GRILL

INGREDIENTS

- 2 lbs. thinly sliced chicken breast
- 1 large red bell pepper
- 1 large onion
- 1 large orange bell pepper.

Seasoning mix:

- 2 tbsp. oil
- ½ tbsp. onion powder
- ½ tbsp. granulated garlic
- 1 tbsp. salt

DIRECTIONS

1. Preheat the grill to 450 degrees.
2. Mix the seasonings and oil.
3. Add the chicken slices to the mix.
4. Line a large pan with a non-stick baking sheet.
5. Let the pan heat for 10 minutes.
6. Place the chicken, peppers, and other vegetables in the grill.
7. Grill for 10 minutes or until the chicken is cooked.
8. Remove it from the grill and serve with warm tortillas and vegetables.

Nutritions: Carbohydrates: 5g Protein: 29g Fat: 6g Sodium: 360mg Cholesterol: 77mg.

23. SMOKED CORNISH CHICKEN IN WOOD PELLETS

INGREDIENTS

- 6 cornish hens
- 2-3 tbsp. canola or avocado oil
- 6 tbsp. spice mix.

DIRECTIONS

1. Preheat your wood pellet grill to 275 degrees.
2. Rub the whole hen with oil and the spice mix. Use both of these ingredients liberally.
3. Place the breast area of the hen on the grill and smoke for 30 minutes.
4. Flip the hen so the breast side is facing up. Increase the temperature to 400 degrees.
5. Cook until the temperature goes down to 165 degrees.
6. Pull it out and leave it for 10 minutes.
7. Serve warm with a side dish of your choice.

Nutritions: Carbohydrates: 1g Protein: 57g Fat: 50g Sodium: 165mg Cholesterol: 337mg.

CHAPTER 5. BEEF RECIPES

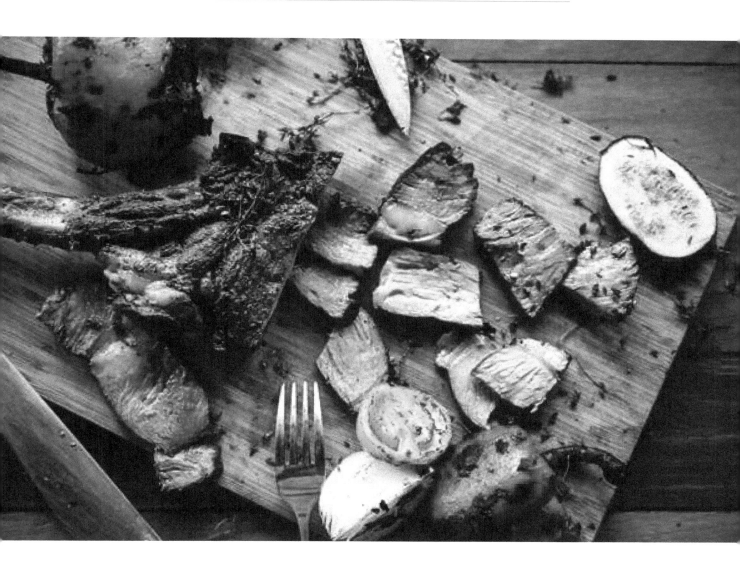

24. TRAEGER BEEF JERKY

INGREDIENTS

- 3 pounds sirloin steaks
- 2 cups soy sauce
- 1 cup pineapple juice
- 1/2 cup brown sugar
- 2 tbsp. sriracha
- 2 tbsp. hoisin
- 2 tbsp. red pepper flake
- 2 tbsp. rice wine vinegar
- 2 tbsp. onion powder.

DIRECTIONS

1. Mix the marinade in a zip lock bag and add the beef. Mix until well coated and remove as much air as possible.
2. Place the bag in a fridge and let marinate overnight or for 6 hours. Remove the bag from the fridge an hour prior to cooking.
3. Startup the Traeger and set it on the smoking settings or at 190°F.
4. Lay the meat on the grill leaving a half-inch space between the pieces. Let cool for 5 hours and turn after 2 hours.
5. Remove from the grill and let cool. Serve or refrigerate.

Nutritions: Calories: 309 Fat: 7g Carbohydrates: 20g Protein: 34g Fiber: 1g.

25. TRAEGER SMOKED BEEF ROAST

INGREDIENTS

- 1-3/4 pounds beef sirloin tip roast
- 1/2 cup barbeque rub
- 2 bottles of amber beer
- 1 bottle BBQ sauce.

DIRECTIONS

1. Turn the Traeger onto the smoke setting.
2. Rub the beef with barbeque rub until well coated, then place on the grill. Let smoke for 4 hours while flipping every 1 hour.
3. Transfer the beef to a pan and add the beer. The beef should be 1/2 way covered.
4. Braise the beef until fork tender. It will take 3 hours on the stovetop and 60 minutes on the instant pot.
5. Remove the beef from the ban and reserve 1 cup of the cooking liquid.
6. Use 2 forks to shred the beef into small pieces, then return to the pan with the reserved braising liquid. Add BBQ sauce and stir well, then keep warm until serving. You can also reheat if it gets cold.

Nutritions: Calories: 829 Fat: 18g Carbohydrates: 4g Protein: 86g Fiber: 0g.

26. BACON-SWISS CHEESESTEAK MEATLOAF

INGREDIENTS

- 1 tablespoon canola oil
- 2 garlic cloves, finely chopped
- 1 medium onion, finely chopped
- 1 poblano chile, stemmed, seeded, and finely chopped
- 2 pounds extra-lean ground beef
- 2 tablespoons Montreal steak seasoning
- 1 tablespoon A.1. Steak Sauce
- ½ pound bacon, cooked and crumbled
- 2 cups shredded Swiss cheese
- 1 egg, beaten
- 2 cups breadcrumbs
- ½ cup Tiger Sauce.

DIRECTIONS

1. On your stove top, heat the canola oil in a medium sauté pan over medium-high heat. Add the garlic, onion, and poblano, and sauté for 3 to 5 minutes, or until the onion is just barely translucent.
2. Supply your smoker with wood pellets and follow the manufacturer's specific start-up procedure. Preheat, with the lid closed, to 225°F.
3. In a large bowl, combine the sautéed vegetables, ground beef, steak seasoning, steak sauce, bacon, Swiss cheese, egg, and breadcrumbs. Mix with your hands until well incorporated, then shape into a loaf.
4. Put the meatloaf in a cast-iron skillet and place it on the grill. Insert meat thermometer inserted in the loaf reads 165°F.
5. Top with the meatloaf with the Tiger Sauce, remove from the grill and let rest for about 10 minutes before serving.

Nutritions: Calories: 120 Fat: 2g Carbohydrates: 0g Protein: 23g Fiber: 0g.

27. LONDON BROIL

INGREDIENTS

- 1 (1½- to 2-pound) London broil or top round steak
- ¼ cup soy sauce
- 2 tablespoons white wine
- 2 tablespoons extra-virgin olive oil
- ¼ cup chopped scallions
- 2 tablespoons packed brown sugar
- 2 garlic cloves, minced
- 2 teaspoons red pepper flakes
- 1 teaspoon freshly ground black pepper.

DIRECTIONS

1. Using a meat mallet, pound the steak lightly all over on both sides to break down its fibers and tenderize. You are not trying to pound down the thickness.
2. In a medium bowl, make the marinade by combining the soy sauce, white wine, olive oil, scallions, brown sugar, garlic, red pepper flakes, and black pepper.
3. Put the steak in a shallow plastic container with a lid and pour the marinade over the meat. Cover and refrigerate for 4 hours.
4. Supply your smoker with wood pellets and follow the manufacturer's specific start-up procedure. Preheat, with the lid closed, to 350°F.
5. Place the steak directly on the grill, close the lid, and smoke for 6 minutes. Flip, then smoke with the lid closed for 6 to 10 minutes more, or until a meat thermometer inserted in the meat reads 130°F for medium-rare.
6. The meat's temperature will rise by about 5 degrees while it rests.

Nutritions: Calories: 316 Fat: 3g Carbohydrates: 0g Protein: 54g Fiber: 0g.

28. FRENCH ONION BURGERS

INGREDIENTS

- 1-pound lean ground beef
- 1 tablespoon minced garlic
- 1 teaspoon Better Than Bouillon Beef Base
- 1 teaspoon dried chives
- 1 teaspoon freshly ground black pepper
- 8 slices Gruyère cheese, divided
- ½ cup soy sauce
- 1 tablespoon extra-virgin olive oil
- 1 teaspoon liquid smoke
- 3 medium onions, cut into thick slices (do not separate the rings)
- 1 loaf French bread, cut into 8 slices
- 4 slices provolone cheese.

DIRECTIONS

1. In a large bowl, mix the ground beef, minced garlic, beef base, chives, and pepper until well blended.
2. Divide the meat mixture and shape into 8 thin burger patties.
3. Top each of 4 patties with one slice of Gruyère, then top with the remaining 4 patties to create 4 stuffed burgers.
4. Supply your smoker with wood pellets and follow the manufacturer's specific start-up procedure. Preheat, with the lid closed, to 425°F.
5. Arrange the burgers directly on one side of the grill, close the lid, and smoke for 10 minutes. Flip and smoke with the lid closed for 10 to 15 minutes more, or until a meat thermometer inserted in the burgers reads 160°F. Add another Gruyère slice to the burgers during the last 5 minutes of smoking to melt.
6. Meanwhile, in a small bowl, combine the soy sauce, olive oil, and liquid smoke.
7. Arrange the onion slices on the grill and baste on both sides with the soy sauce mixture. Smoke with the lid closed for 20 minutes, flipping halfway through.
8. Lightly toast the French bread slices on the grill. Layer each of 4 slices with a burger patty, a slice of provolone cheese, and some of the smoked onions. Top each with another slice of toasted French bread. Serve immediately.

Nutritions: Calories: 704 Fat: 43g Carbohydrates: 28g Protein: 49g Fiber: 2g.

29. BEEF SHOULDER CLOD

INGREDIENTS

- ½ cup sea salt
- ½ cup freshly ground black pepper
- 1 tablespoon red pepper flakes
- 1 tablespoon minced garlic
- 1 tablespoon cayenne pepper
- 1 tablespoon smoked paprika
- 1 (13- to 15-pound) beef shoulder clod.

DIRECTIONS

1. Combine spices.
2. Generously apply it to the beef shoulder.
3. Supply your smoker with wood pellets and follow the manufacturer's specific start-up procedure. Preheat, with the lid closed, to 250°F.
4. Put the meat on the grill grate, close the lid, and smoke for 12 to 16 hours, or until a meat thermometer inserted deeply into the beef reads 195°F. You may need to cover the clod with aluminum foil toward the end of smoking to prevent overbrowning.
5. Let the meat rest and serve.

Nutritions: Calories: 290 Fat: 22g Carbohydrates: 0g Protein: 20g Fiber: 0g.

30. CORNED BEEF AND CABBAGE

INGREDIENTS

- 1 gallon water
- 1 (3- to 4-pound) point cut corned beef brisket with pickling spice packet
- 1 tablespoon freshly ground black pepper
- 1 tablespoon garlic powder
- ½ cup molasses
- 1 teaspoon ground mustard
- 1 head green cabbage
- 4 tablespoons (½ stick) butter
- 2 tablespoons rendered bacon fat
- 1 chicken bouillon cube, crushed.

DIRECTIONS

1. Refrigerate overnight, changing the water as often as you remember to do so—ideally, every 3 hours while you're awake—to soak out some of the curing salt originally added.
2. Supply your smoker with wood pellets and follow the manufacturer's specific start-up procedure. Preheat, with the lid closed, to 275°F.
3. Remove the meat from the brining liquid, pat it dry, and generously rub with the black pepper and garlic powder.
4. Put the seasoned corned beef directly on the grill, fat-side up, close the lid, and grill for 2 hours. Remove from the grill when done.
5. In a small bowl, combine the molasses and ground mustard and pour half of this mixture into the bottom of a disposable aluminum pan.
6. Transfer the meat to the pan, fat-side up, and pour the remaining molasses mixture on top, spreading it evenly over the meat. Cover tightly with aluminum foil.
7. Transfer the pan to the grill, close the lid, and continue smoking the corned beef for 2 to 3 hours or until a meat thermometer inserted in the thickest part reads 185°F.
8. Rest meat
9. Serve.

Nutritions: Calories: 295 Fat: 17g Carbohydrates: 19g Protein: 18g Fiber: 6g.

31. REVERSE SEARED FLANK STEAK

INGREDIENTS

- 3 pound flank steaks
- 1 tbsp. salt
- 1/2 tbsp. onion powder
- 1/4 tbsp. garlic powder
- 1/2 black pepper, coarsely ground.

DIRECTIONS

1. Preheat the Traeger to 225°F.
2. Add the steaks and rub them generously with the rub mixture.
3. Place the steak
4. Let cook until its internal temperature is 100°F under your desired temperature. 115°F for rare, 125°F for the medium rear, and 135°F for medium.
5. Wrap the steak with foil and raise the grill temperature to high. Place back the steak and grill for 3 minutes on each side.
6. Pat with butter and serve when hot.

Nutritions: Calories: 112 Fat: 5g Carbohydrates: 1g Protein: 16g Fiber: 0g.

32. TRAEGER NEW YORK STRIP

INGREDIENTS

- 3 New York strips
- Salt and pepper.

DIRECTIONS

1. If the steak is in the fridge, remove it 30 minutes prior to cooking.
2. Preheat the Traeger to 450°F.
3. Meanwhile, season the steak generously with salt and pepper. Place it on the grill and let it cook for 5 minutes per side or until the internal temperature reaches 128°F.
4. Rest for 10 minutes.

Nutritions: Calories: 198 Fat: 14g Carbohydrates: 0g Protein: 17g Fiber: 0g.

33. TRAEGER STUFFED PEPPERS

INGREDIENTS

- 3 bell peppers, sliced in halves
- 1 pound ground beef, lean
- 1 onion, chopped
- 1/2 tbsp. red pepper flakes
- 1/2 tbsp. salt
- 1/4 tbsp. pepper
- 1/2 tbsp. garlic powder
- 1/2 tbsp. onion powder
- 1/2 cup white rice
- 15 oz. stewed tomatoes
- 8 oz. tomato sauce
- 6 cups cabbage, shredded
- 1-1/2 cup water
- 2 cups cheddar cheese.

DIRECTIONS

1. Arrange the pepper halves on a baking tray and set aside.
2. Preheat your grill to 325°F.
3. Brown the meat in a large skillet. Add onions, pepper flakes, salt, pepper garlic, and onion and cook until the meat is well cooked.
4. Add rice, stewed tomatoes, tomato sauce, cabbage, and water. Cover and simmer until the rice is well cooked, the cabbage is tender, and there is no water in the rice.
5. Place the cooked beef mixture in the pepper halves and top with cheese.
6. Place in the grill and cook for 30 minutes.
7. Serve immediately and enjoy it.

Nutritions: Calories: 422 Fat: 22g Carbohydrates: 24g Protein: 34g Fiber: 5g.

34. TRAEGER KALBI BEEF SHORT RIBS

INGREDIENTS

- 1/2 cup soy sauce
- 1/2 cup brown sugar
- 1/8 cup rice wine
- 2 tbsp. minced garlic
- 1 tbsp. sesame oil
- 1/8 cup onion, finely grated
- 2-1/2 pound beef short ribs, thinly sliced.

DIRECTIONS

1. Mix soy sauce, sugar, rice wine, garlic, sesame oil, and onion in a medium mixing bowl.
2. Add the beef to the bowl and cover it in the marinade. Cover the bowl with a plastic wrap and refrigerate for 6 hours.
3. Heat your Traeger to high and ensure the grill is well heated.
4. Place on grill and close the lid, ensuring you don't lose any heat.
5. Cook for 4 minutes, flip, and cook for 4 more minutes on the other side.
6. Remove the meat and serve with rice and veggies of choice. Enjoy.

Nutritions: Calories: 355 Fat: 10g Carbohydrates: 22g Protein: 28g Fiber: 0g.

35. TRAEGER BEEF SHORT RIB LOLLIPOP

INGREDIENTS

- 4 beef short rib lollipops
- BBQ Rub
- BBQ Sauce.

DIRECTIONS

1. Preheat your Traeger to 275°F.
2. Season the short ribs with BBQ rub and place them on the grill.
3. Cook for 4 hours while turning occasionally until the meat is tender.
4. Apply the sauce to the meat in the last 30 minutes of cooking.
5. Serve and enjoy.

Nutritions: Calories: 265 Fat: 19g Carbohydrates: 1g Protein: 22g Fiber: 0g.

CHAPTER 6. PORK RECIPES

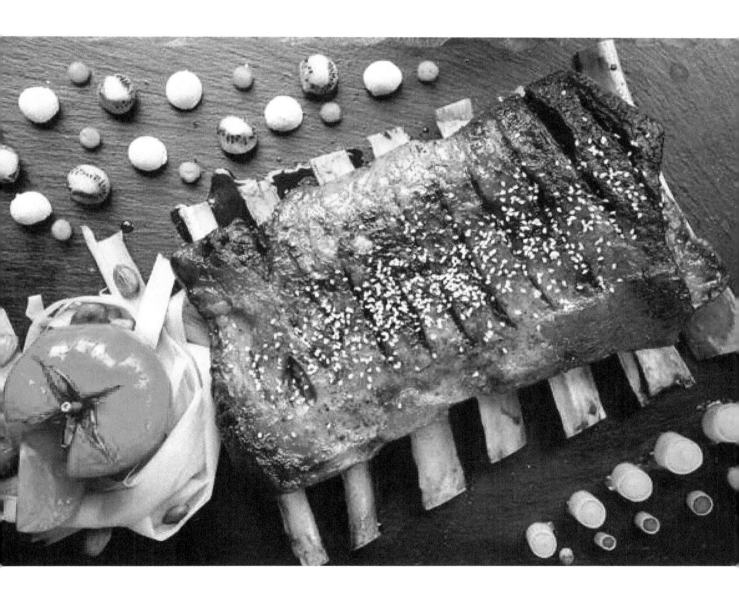

36. SMOKED BABY BACK RIBS

INGREDIENTS

- 3 racks baby back ribs
- Salt and pepper to taste.

DIRECTIONS

1. Clean the ribs by removing the extra membrane that covers it. Pat dry the ribs with a clean paper towel. Season the baby back ribs with salt and pepper to taste. Allow to rest in the fridge for at least 4 hours before cooking.
2. Once ready to cook, fire the Traeger Grill to 225°F. Use hickory wood pellets when cooking the ribs. Close the lid and preheat for 15 minutes.
3. Place the ribs on the grill grate and cook for two hours. Carefully flipping the ribs halfway through the cooking time for even cooking.

Nutritions: Calories: 1037 Protein: 92.5g Carbs: 1.4g Fat: 73.7g Sugar: 0.2g.

37. SMOKED APPLE PORK TENDERLOIN

INGREDIENTS

- ½ cup apple juice
- 3 tablespoons honey
- 3 tablespoons Traeger Pork and Poultry Rub
- ¼ cup brown sugar
- 2 tablespoons thyme leaves
- ½ tablespoons black pepper
- 2 pork tenderloin roasts, skin removed.

DIRECTIONS

1. In a bowl, mix together the apple juice, honey, pork and poultry rub, brown sugar, thyme, and black pepper. Whisk to mix everything.
2. Add the pork loins into the marinade and allow it to soak for 3 hours in the fridge.
3. Once ready to cook, fire the Traeger Grill to 225°F. Use hickory wood pellets when cooking the ribs. Close the lid and preheat for 15 minutes.
4. Place the marinated pork loin on the grill grate and cook until the temperature registers to 145°F. Cook for 2 to 3 hours on low heat.
5. Meanwhile, place the marinade in a saucepan. Place the saucepan in the grill and allow to simmer until the sauce has reduced.
6. Before taking the meat out, baste the pork with the reduced marinade.
7. Allow to rest for 10 minutes before slicing.

Nutritions: Calories: 203 Protein: 26.4g Carbs: 15.4g Fat: 3.6g Sugar: 14.6g.

38. COMPETITION STYLE BARBECUE PORK RIBS

INGREDIENTS

- 2 racks of St. Louis-style ribs
- 1 cup Traeger Pork and Poultry Rub
- 1/8 cup brown sugar
- 4 tablespoons butter
- 4 tablespoons agave
- 1 bottle Traeger Sweet and Heat BARBECUE Sauce.

DIRECTIONS

1. Place the ribs on the work surface and remove the thin film of connective tissues covering it. In a smaller bowl, combine the Traeger Pork and Poultry Rub, brown sugar, butter, and agave. Mix until well combined.
2. Massage the rub onto the ribs and allow them to rest in the fridge for at least 2 hours.
3. When ready to cook, fire the Traeger Grill to 225°F. Use desired wood pellets when cooking the ribs. Close the lid and preheat for 15 minutes.
4. Place the ribs on the grill grate and close the lid. Smoke for 1 hour and 30 minutes. Make sure to flip the ribs halfway through the cooking time.
5. Ten minutes before the cooking time ends, brush the ribs with Barbecue sauce.
6. Remove from the grill and allow to rest before slicing.

Nutritions: Calories: 399 Protein: 47.2g Carbs: 3.5g Fat: 20.5g Sugar: 2.3g.

39. SMOKED SPARE RIBS

INGREDIENTS

- 2 (2- or 3-pound) racks spare ribs
- 2 tablespoons yellow mustard
- 1 batch Sweet Brown Sugar Rub
- ¼ cup Bill's Best BBQ Sauce.

DIRECTIONS

1. Supply your smoker with wood pellets and follow the manufacturer's specific start-up procedure. With lid closed, preheat grill
2. The membrane must be removed. This can be done by cutting just through the membrane in an X pattern and working a paper towel between the membrane and the ribs to pull it off.
3. Coat the ribs on both sides with mustard and season with the rub. Work rub onto meat.
4. Put the ribs on the grill and smoke until their internal temperature reaches between 190°F and 200°F.
5. Drizzle barbeque sauce.
6. Increase the grill's temperature to 300°F and continue to cook the ribs for 15 minutes more.
7. Remove the racks from the grill, cut them into individual ribs, and serve immediately.

Nutritions: Calories: 318 Fat: 24g Carbohydrates: 0g Protein: 23g Fiber: 0g.

40. SWEET SMOKED COUNTRY RIBS

INGREDIENTS

- 2 pounds country-style ribs
- 1 batch Sweet Brown Sugar Rub
- 2 tablespoons light brown sugar
- 1 cup Pepsi or another cola
- ¼ cup Bill's Best BBQ Sauce.

DIRECTIONS

1. Supply your smoker with wood pellets and follow the manufacturer's specific start-up procedure. With the lid closed, preheat the grill until the temperature is 180 degrees.
2. Sprinkle the ribs with the rub and use your hands to work the rub into the meat.
3. Place the ribs directly on the grill grate and smoke for 3 hours.
4. Remove the ribs from the grill and place them on enough aluminum foil to wrap them completely. Dust the brown sugar over the ribs.
5. Increase the grill's temperature to 300°F.
6. Fold in three sides of the foil around the ribs and add the cola. Fold in the last side, completely enclosing the ribs and liquid. Return the ribs to the grill and cook for 45 minutes.
7. Remove the ribs from the foil and place them on the grill grate. Baste all sides of the ribs with barbecue sauce. Cook for 15 minutes more to caramelize the sauce.
8. Remove the ribs from the grill and serve immediately.

Nutritions: Calories: 230 Fat: 17g Carbohydrates: 0g Protein: 20g Fiber: 0g.

41. CLASSIC PULLED PORK

INGREDIENTS

- 1 (6- to 8-pound) bone-in pork shoulder
- 2 tablespoons yellow mustard
- 1 batch Not-Just-for-Pork Rub.

DIRECTIONS

1. Supply your smoker with wood pellets and follow the manufacturer's specific start-up procedure.
2. Coat the pork shoulder all over with mustard and season it with the rub.
3. Place the shoulder on the grill grate and smoke until its internal temperature reaches 195°F.
4. Pull the shoulder from the grill and wrap it completely in aluminum foil or butcher paper. Place it in a cooler, cover the cooler, and let it rest for 1 or 2 hours.
5. Remove the pork shoulder from the cooler and unwrap it. Remove the shoulder bone and pull the pork apart using just your fingers. Serve immediately as desired. Leftovers are encouraged.

Nutritions: Calories: 414 Fat: 29g Carbohydrates: 1g Protein: 38g Fiber: 0g.

42. RUB-INJECTED PORK SHOULDER

INGREDIENTS

- 1 (6- to 8-pound) bone-in pork shoulder
- 2 cups Tea Injectable made with Not-Just-for-Pork Rub
- 2 tablespoons yellow mustard
- 1 batch Not-Just-for-Pork Rub.

DIRECTIONS

1. Supply your smoker with wood pellets and follow the manufacturer's specific start-up procedure.
2. Inject the pork shoulder throughout with the tea injectable.
3. Coat the pork shoulder all over with mustard and season it with the rub. Work rub onto
4. Place the shoulder directly on the grill grate and smoke until its internal temperature reaches 160°F, and a dark bark has formed on the exterior.
5. Pull the shoulder from the grill and wrap it completely in aluminum foil or butcher paper.
6. Increase the grill's temperature to 350°F.
7. Return the pork shoulder to the grill and cook until its internal temperature reaches 195°F.
8. Pull the shoulder from the grill and place it in a cooler. Cover the cooler and let the pork rest for 1 or 2 hours.
9. Remove the pork shoulder from the cooler and unwrap it. Remove the shoulder bone and pull the pork apart using just your fingers. Serve immediately.

Nutritions: Calories: 257 Fat: 15g Carbohydrates: 0g Protein: 29g Fiber: 0g.

43. MAPLE-SMOKED PORK CHOPS

INGREDIENTS

- 4 (8-ounce) pork chops, bone-in or boneless (I use boneless)
- Salt
- Freshly ground black pepper.

DIRECTIONS

1. Supply your smoker with wood pellets and follow the manufacturer's specific start-up procedure.
2. Drizzle pork chop with salt and pepper to season.
3. Place the chops directly on the grill grate and smoke for 30 minutes.
4. Increase the grill's temperature to 350°F. Continue to cook the chops until their internal temperature reaches 145°F.
5. Remove the pork chops from the grill and let them rest for 5 minutes before serving.

Nutritions: Calories: 130 Fat: 12g Carbohydrates: 3g Protein: 20g Fiber: 0g.

44. APPLE-SMOKED PORK TENDERLOIN

INGREDIENTS

- 2 (1-pound) pork tenderloins
- 1 batch Not-Just-for-Pork Rub.

DIRECTIONS

1. Supply your smoker with wood pellets and follow the manufacturer's specific start-up procedure. Preheat the grill
2. Generously season the tenderloins with the rub. W
3. Put tenderloins on the grill and smoke for 4 or 5 hours, until their internal temperature reaches 145°F.
4. The tenderloins must be put out of the grill and let it rest for 5-10 minutes, then begin slicing into thin pieces before serving

Nutritions: Calories: 180 Fat: 8g Carbohydrates: 3g Protein: 24g Fiber: 0g.

45. TERIYAKI PORK TENDERLOIN

INGREDIENTS

- 2 (1-pound) pork tenderloins
- 1 batch Easy Teriyaki Marinade
- Smoked salt.

DIRECTIONS

1. In a large zip-top bag, combine the tenderloins and marinade. Seal the bag, turn to coat, and refrigerate the pork for at least 30 minutes—I recommend up to overnight.
2. Supply your smoker with wood pellets and follow the manufacturer's specific start-up procedure. Preheat the grill, with the lid closed, to 180°F.
3. As you get the tenderloins from the marinade, begin seasoning them with smoked salt
4. Place the tenderloins directly on the grill grate and smoke for 1 hour.
5. Increase the grill's temperature to 300°F and continue to cook until the pork's internal temperature reaches 145°F.
6. With the tenderloins removed from the grill, let it cool for at least 5-10 minutes before slicing and serving.

Nutritions: Calories: 110 Fat: 3g Carbohydrates: 2g Protein: 18g Fiber: 0g.

46. SMOKED APPLE BARBECUE RIBS

INGREDIENTS

- 2 racks St. Louis-style ribs
- ¼ cup Traeger Big Game Rub
- 1 cup apple juice
- A bottle of Traeger BARBECUE Sauce.

DIRECTIONS

1. Place the ribs on a working surface and remove the film of connective tissues covering it.
2. In another bowl, mix the Game Rub and apple juice until well-combined.
3. Massage the rub onto the ribs and allow them to rest in the fridge for at least 2 hours.
4. When ready to cook, fire the Traeger Grill to 225°F. Use apple wood pellets when cooking the ribs. Close the lid and preheat for 15 minutes.
5. Place the ribs on the grill grate and close the lid. Smoke for 1 hour and 30 minutes. Make sure to flip the ribs halfway through the cooking time.
6. Ten minutes before the cooking time ends, brush the ribs with BARBECUE sauce.
7. Remove from the grill and allow to rest before slicing.

Nutritions: Calories: 337 Protein: 47.1g Carbs: 4.7g Fat: 12.9g Sugar: 4g.

47. CITRUS-BRINED PORK ROAST

INGREDIENTS

- ½ cup salt
- ¼ cup brown sugar
- 3 cloves of garlic, minced
- 2 dried bay leaves
- 6 peppercorns
- 1 lemon, juiced
- ½ teaspoon dried fennel seeds
- ½ teaspoon red pepper flakes
- ½ cup apple juice
- ½ cup orange juice
- 5 pounds pork loin
- 2 tablespoons extra virgin olive oil.

DIRECTIONS

1. In a bowl, combine the salt, brown sugar, garlic, bay leaves, peppercorns, lemon juice, fennel seeds, pepper flakes, apple juice, and orange juice. Mix to form a paste rub.
2. Rub the mixture onto the pork loin and allow it to marinate for at least 2 hours in the fridge. Add in the oil.
3. When ready to cook, fire the Traeger Grill to 300°F. Use apple wood pellets when cooking. Close the lid and preheat for 15 minutes.
4. Place the seasoned pork loin on the grill grate and close the lid. Cook for 45 minutes. Make sure to flip the pork halfway through the cooking time.

Nutritions: Calories: 869 Protein: 97.2g Carbs: 15.2g Fat: 43.9g Sugar: 13g.

48. PINEAPPLE PORK BARBECUE

INGREDIENTS

- 1-pound pork sirloin
- 4 cups pineapple juice
- 3 cloves garlic, minced
- 1 cup carne asada marinade
- 2 tablespoons salt
- 1 teaspoon ground black pepper.

DIRECTIONS

1. Place all ingredients in a bowl. Massage the pork sirloin to coat with all ingredients. Place inside the fridge to marinate for at least 2 hours.
2. When ready to cook, fire the Traeger Grill to 300°F. Use desired wood pellets when cooking the ribs. Close the lid and preheat for 15 minutes.
3. Place the pork sirloin on the grill grate and cook for 45 to 60 minutes. Make sure to flip the pork halfway through the cooking time.
4. At the same time, when you put the pork on the grill grate, place the marinade in a pan and place it inside the smoker. Allow the marinade to cook and reduce.
5. Baste the pork sirloin with the reduced marinade before the cooking time ends.
6. Allow to rest before slicing.

Nutritions: Calories: 347 Protein: 33.4g Carbs: 45.8g Fat: 4.2g Sugar: 36g.

49. BARBECUE SPARERIBS WITH MANDARIN GLAZE

INGREDIENTS

- 3 large spareribs, membrane removed
- 3 tablespoons yellow mustard
- 1 tablespoons Worcestershire sauce
- 1 cup honey
- 1 ½ cup brown sugar
- 13 ounces Traeger Mandarin Glaze
- 1 teaspoon sesame oil
- 1 teaspoon soy sauce
- 1 teaspoon garlic powder.

DIRECTIONS

1. Place the spareribs on a working surface and carefully remove the connective tissue membrane that covers the ribs.
2. In another bowl, mix the rest of the ingredients until well combined. Massage the spice mixture onto the spareribs. Allow to rest in the fridge for at least 3 hours.
3. When ready to cook, fire the Traeger Grill to 300°F. Use hickory wood pellets when cooking the ribs. Close the lid and preheat for 15 minutes.
4. Place the seasoned ribs on the grill grate and cover the lid. Cook for 60 minutes.
5. Once cooked, allow to rest before slicing.

Nutritions: Calories: 1263 Protein: 36.9g Carbs: 110.3g Fat: 76.8g Sugar: 107g.

CHAPTER 7. BURGERS AND SAUSAGES

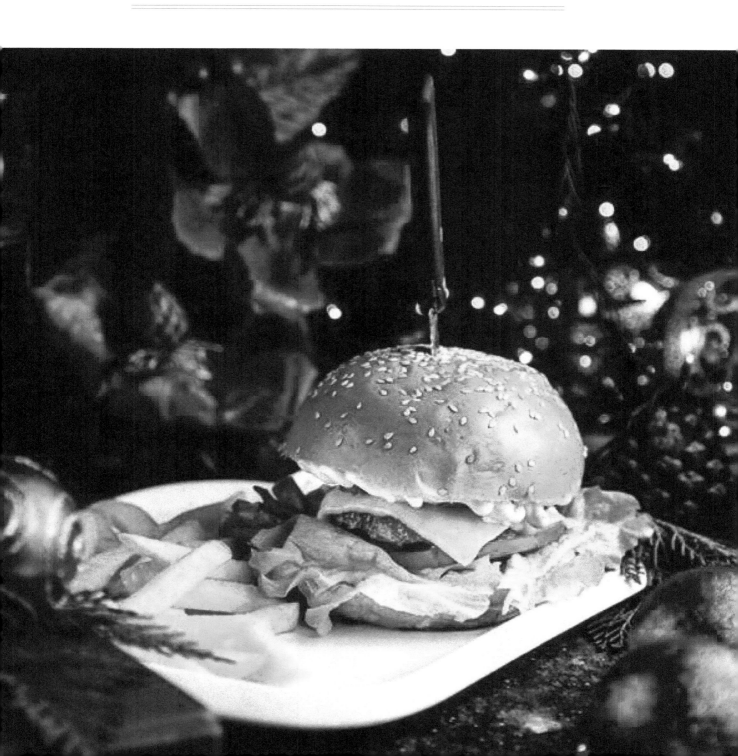

50. BREAKFAST SAUSAGE

INGREDIENTS

- 20/22 millimeter natural sheep casings, rinsed
- Warm water
- 2 lb. ground pork
- Apple butter rub
- Pinch dried marjoram
- 1/2 teaspoon ground cloves
- 1 tablespoon brown sugar
- 1/3 cup ice water
- Pepper to taste.

DIRECTIONS

1. Soak the sheep casings in warm water for 1 hour.
2. In a bowl, mix all the ingredients.
3. Use a mixer set on low speed to combine the ingredients.
4. Cover and refrigerate the mixture for 15 minutes.
5. Insert the casings into the sausage stuffer.
6. Stuff the casings with the ground pork mixture.
7. Twist into five links.
8. Remove bubbles using a pricker.
9. Put the sausages on a baking pan.
10. Refrigerate for 24 hours.
11. Set your wood pellet grill to smoke.
12. Hang the sausages on hooks and put them in the smoking cabinet.
13. Set the temperature to 350 degrees F.
14. Smoke the sausages for 1 hour.
15. Increase the temperature to 425 degrees F.
16. Cook for another 30 minutes.

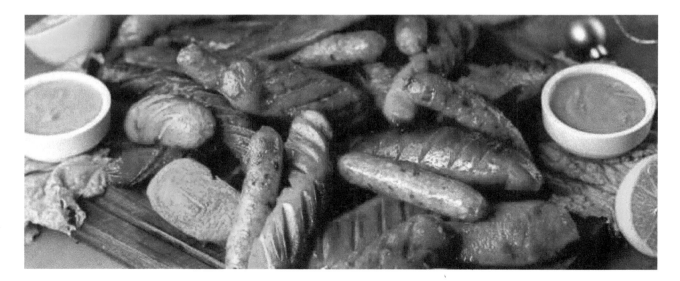

Nutritions: Calories: 220 Fat: 19g Cholesterol: 45mg Carbohydrates: 1g Fiber: 0g Sugars: 1g Protein: 11g.

51. GRILLED STEAK WITH AMERICAN CHEESE SANDWICH

INGREDIENTS

- 1 pound of beef steak.
- 1/2 teaspoon of salt to taste.
- 1/2 teaspoon of pepper to taste.
- 1 tablespoon of Worcestershire sauce.
- 2 tablespoons of butter.
- 1 chopped onion.
- 1/2 chopped green bell pepper.
- Salt and pepper to taste.
- 8 slices of American cheese.
- 8 slices of white bread.
- 4 tablespoons of butter.

DIRECTIONS

1. Turn your Wood Pellet Smoker and Grill to smoke and fire up for about four to five minutes. Set the temperature of the grill to 450 degrees F and let it preheat for about ten to fifteen minutes with its lid closed.
2. Next, place a non-stick skillet on the griddle and preheat for about fifteen minutes until it becomes hot. Once hot, add in the butter and let melt. Once the butter melts, add in the onions and green bell pepper, then cook for about five minutes until they become brown in color; set aside.
3. Next, still using the same pan on the griddle, add in the steak, Worcestershire sauce, salt, and pepper to taste, then cook for about five to six minutes until it is cooked through. Add in the cooked bell pepper mixture; stir to combine, then heat for another three minutes, set aside.
4. Use a sharp knife to slice the bread in half, butter each side, then grill for about three to four minutes with its sides down. To assemble, add slices of cheese on each bread slice, top with the steak mixture, then your favorite toppings, close the sandwich with another bread slice then serve.

Nutritions: Calories: 589 Carbohydrates: 28g Protein: 24g Fat: 41g Fiber: 2g.

52. GRILLED LAMB BURGERS

INGREDIENTS

- 1 1/4 pounds of ground lamb.
- 1 egg
- 1 teaspoon of dried oregano
- 1 teaspoon of dry sherry
- 1 teaspoon of white wine vinegar
- 1/2 teaspoon of crushed red pepper flakes
- 4 minced cloves of garlic
- 1/2 cup of chopped green onions
- 1 tablespoon of chopped minutest
- 2 tablespoons of chopped cilantro
- 2 tablespoons of dry bread crumbs
- 1/8 teaspoon of salt to taste
- 1/4 teaspoon of ground black pepper to taste
- 5 hamburger buns.

DIRECTIONS

1. Preheat a Wood Pellet Smoker or Grill to 350-450 degrees F, then grease it grates. Using a large mixing bowl, add in all the ingredients on the list aside from the buns, then mix properly to combine with clean hands. Make about five patties out of the mixture, then set aside.
2. Place the lamb patties on the preheated grill and cook for about seven to nine minutes, turning only once until an inserted thermometer reads 160 degrees F. Serve the lamb burgers on the hamburger, add your favorite toppings and enjoy.

Nutritions: Calories: 376 Fat: 18.5g Fiber: 1.6g Carbohydrates: 25.4g Protein: 25.5g.

53. GROUND TURKEY BURGERS

INGREDIENTS

- 1 beaten egg
- 2/3 cup of bread crumbs.
- 1/2 cup of chopped celery
- 1/4 cup of chopped onion
- 1 tablespoon of minced parsley
- 1 teaspoon of Worcestershire sauce
- 1 teaspoon of dried oregano
- 1/2 teaspoon of salt to taste
- 1/4 teaspoon of pepper
- 1-1/4 pounds of lean ground turkey
- 6 hamburger buns
- Optional topping
- 1 sliced tomato
- 1 sliced onion
- Lettuce leaves.

DIRECTIONS

1. Using a small mixing bowl, add in all the ingredients on the list aside from the turkey and buns, then mix properly to combine. Add in the ground turkey, then mix everything to combine. Feel free to use clean hands for this. Make about six patties of the mixture, then set aside.
2. Preheat your Wood Pellet Smoker and Grill to 375 degrees F, place the turkey patties on the grill and grill for about forty-five minutes until its internal temperature reads 165 degrees F. to assemble, use a knife to split the bun into two, top with the prepared burger and your favorite topping then close with another half of the buns, serve.

Nutritions: Calories: 293 Fat: 11g Carbohydrates: 27g Fiber: 4g Protein: 22g.

54. BARBECUE SHREDDED BEEF BURGER

INGREDIENTS

- 3 pounds of boneless chuck roast.
- Salt to taste
- Pepper to taste
- 2 tablespoons of minced garlic
- 1 cup of chopped onion
- 28 oz. of barbeque sauce
- 6 buns.

DIRECTIONS

1. Set the temperature of the Wood Pellet Smoker and Grill to 250 degrees F, then preheat for about fifteen minutes with its lid closed. Use a knife to trim off the excess fat present on the roast, then place the meat on the preheated grill. Grill the roast for about three and a half hours until it attains an internal temperature of 160 degrees F.
2. Next, place the chuck roast in an aluminum foil, add in the garlic, onion, barbeque sauce, salt, and pepper, then stir to coat. Place the roast bake on the grill and cook for another one and a half hour until an inserted thermometer reads 204 degrees F.
3. Once cooked, let the meat cool for a few minutes, then shred with a fork. Fill the buns with the shredded beef, then serve.

Nutritions: Calories: 593 Fat: 31g Carbohydrates: 34g Fiber: 1g Protein: 44g.

55. GRILLED PORK BURGERS

INGREDIENTS

- 1 beaten egg
- 3/4 cup of soft breadcrumbs
- 3/4 cup of grated parmesan cheese
- 1 tablespoon of dried parsley
- 2 teaspoons of dried basil
- 1/2 teaspoon of salt to taste
- 1/2 teaspoon of garlic powder
- 1/4 teaspoon of pepper to taste
- 2 pounds of ground pork
- 6 hamburger buns
- Toppings
- Lettuce leaves
- Sliced tomato
- Sliced sweet onion.

DIRECTIONS

1. Using a large mixing bowl, add in the egg, bread crumbs, cheese, parsley, basil, garlic powder, salt, and pepper to taste, then mix properly to combine. Add in the ground pork, then mix properly to combine using clean hands. Form about six patties with the mixture, then set aside.
2. Next, set a Wood Pellet smoker and grill to smoke (250 degrees F), then let it fire up for about five minutes. Place the patties on the grill and smoke for about thirty minutes. Flip the patties over, increase the temperature of the grill to 300 degrees F, then grill the patties for a few minutes until an inserted thermometer reads 160 degrees F.
3. Serve the pork burgers on the buns, lettuce, tomato, and onion.

Nutritions: Calories: 522 Fat: 28g Carbohydrates: 28g Fiber: 2g Protein: 38g.

CHAPTER 8. VEGETABLES RECIPES

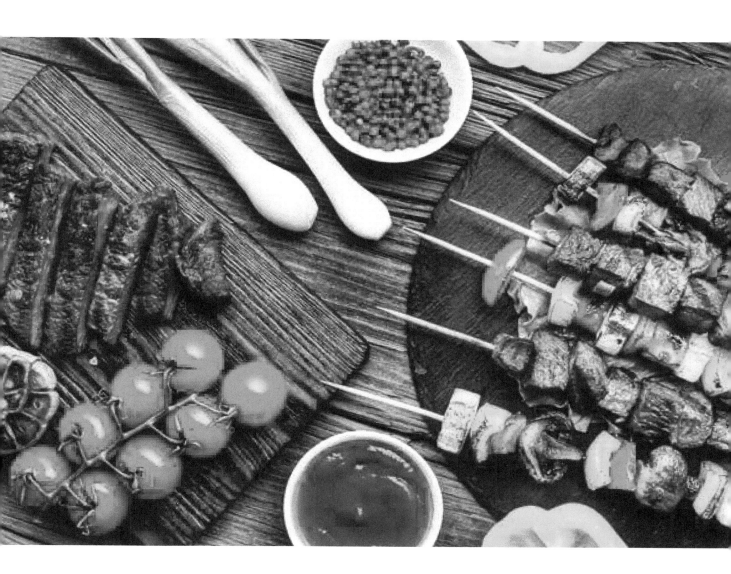

56. SMOKEY ROASTED CAULIFLOWER

INGREDIENTS

- 1 head cauliflower
- 1 cup parmesan cheese

Spice Ingredients:

- 1 tbsp. olive oil
- 2 cloves garlic, chopped
- 1 tsp. kosher salt
- 1 tsp. smoked paprika.

DIRECTIONS

1. Preheat pellet grill to 180°F. If applicable, set smoke setting to high.
2. Cut cauliflower into bite-size flowerets and place in a grill basket. Place basket on the grill grate and smoke for an hour.
3. Mix spice Ingredients: In a small bowl while the cauliflower is smoking. Remove cauliflower from the grill after an hour and let cool.
4. Change grill temperature to 425°F. After the cauliflower has cooled, put cauliflower in a resealable bag, and pour marinade in the bag. Toss to combine in the bag.
5. Place cauliflower back in a grill basket and return to grill. Roast in the grill basket for 10-12 minutes or until the outsides begin to get crispy and golden brown.
6. Remove from grill and transfer to a serving dish. Sprinkle parmesan cheese over the cauliflower and rest for a few minutes so the cheese can melt. Serve and enjoy!

Nutritions: Calories: 70 Fat: 35g Cholesterol: 0 Carbohydrates: 7g Fiber: 3g Sugar: 3g Protein: 3g.

57. SMOKED DEVILED EGGS

INGREDIENTS

- 6 large eggs
- 1 slice bacon
- 1/4 cup mayonnaise
- 1 tsp. Dijon mustard
- 1 tsp. apple cider vinegar
- 1/4 tsp. paprika
- Pinch of kosher salt
- 1 tbsp. chives, chopped.

DIRECTIONS

1. Preheat pellet grill to 180°F and turn smoke setting on, if applicable.
2. Bring a pot of water to a boil. Add eggs and hard boil eggs for about 12 minutes.
3. Remove eggs from the pot and place them into an ice-water bath. Once eggs have cooled completely, peel them and slice in half lengthwise.
4. Place sliced eggs on grill, yolk side up. Smoke for 30 to 45 minutes, depending on how much smoky flavor you want.
5. While eggs smoke, cook bacon until it's crispy.
6. Remove eggs from the grill and allow to cool on a plate.
7. Remove the yolks and place all of them in a small bowl. Place the egg whites on a plate.
8. Mash yolks with a fork and add mayonnaise, mustard, apple cider vinegar, paprika, and salt. Stir until combined.
9. Spoon a scoop of yolk mixture back into each egg white.
10. Sprinkle paprika, chives, and crispy bacon bits to garnish. Serve and enjoy!

Nutritions: Calories: 140 Fat: 12g Cholesterol: 190mg Carbohydrates: 1g Fiber: 0 Sugar: 0 Protein: 6g.

58. CRISPY MAPLE BACON BRUSSELS SPROUTS

INGREDIENTS

- 1 lb. Brussels sprouts, trimmed and quartered
- 6 slices thick-cut bacon
- 3 tbsp. maple syrup
- 1 tsp. olive oil
- 1/2 tsp. kosher salt
- 1/2 tsp. ground black pepper.

DIRECTIONS

1. Preheat pellet grill to 425°F.
2. Cut bacon into 1/2 inch thick slices.
3. Place Brussels sprouts in a single layer in the cast iron skillet. Drizzle with olive oil and maple syrup, then toss to coat. Sprinkle bacon slices on top, then season with kosher salt and black pepper.
4. Place skillet in the pellet grill and roast for about 40 to 45 minutes, or until the Brussels sprouts are caramelized and brown.
5. Remove skillet from grill and allow Brussels sprouts to cool for about 5 to 10 minutes. Serve and enjoy!

Nutritions: Calories: 175.3 Fat: 12.1g Cholesterol: 6.6mg Carbohydrates: 13.6g Fiber: 2.9g Sugar: 7.6g Protein: 4.8g.

59. SWEET JALAPEÑO CORNBREAD

INGREDIENTS

- 2/3 cup margarine, softened
- 2/3 cup white sugar
- 2 cups cornmeal
- 1 1/3 cups all-purpose flour
- 4 tsp. baking powder
- 1 tsp. kosher salt
- 3 eggs
- 1 2/3 cups milk
- 1 cup jalapeños, deseeded and chopped
- Butter to line baking dish.

DIRECTIONS

1. Preheat pellet grill to 400°F.
2. Beat margarine and sugar together in a medium-sized bowl until smooth.
3. In another bowl, combine cornmeal, flour, baking powder, and salt.
4. In a third bowl, combine and whisk eggs and milk.
5. Pour 1/3 of the milk mixture and 1/3 of the flour mixture into the margarine mixture at a time, whisking just until mixed after each pour.
6. Once thoroughly combined, stir in chopped jalapeño.
7. Lightly butter the bottom of the baking dish. Pour cornbread mixture evenly into the baking dish.
8. Place dish on grill grates and close the lid. Cook for about 23-25 minutes, or until thoroughly cooked. The way to test is by inserting a toothpick into the center of the cornbread - it should come out clean once removed.
9. Remove dish from the grill and allow to rest for 10 minutes before slicing and serving.

Nutritions: Calories: 160 Fat: 6g Cholesterol: 15mg Carbohydrates: 25g Fiber: 10g Sugar: 0.5g Protein: 3g.

60. GRILLED BROCCOLI

INGREDIENTS

- 2 cups of broccoli, fresh
- 1 tablespoon of canola oil
- 1 teaspoon of lemon pepper.

DIRECTIONS

1. Place the grill; grate inside the unit, and close the hood.
2. Preheat the grill by turning at high for 10 minutes.
3. Meanwhile, mix broccoli with lemon pepper and canola oil.
4. Toss well to coat the Ingredients: thoroughly.
5. Place it on a grill grade once add food appears.
6. Lock the unit and cook for 3 minutes at medium.
7. Take out and serve.

Nutritions: Calories: 96 Total Fat: 7.3g Saturated Fat: 0.5g Cholesterol: 0mg Sodium: 30mg Total Carbohydrates: 6.7g Dietary Fiber: 2.7g Total Sugars: 1.6g Protein: 2.7g.

61. SMOKED HEALTHY CABBAGE

INGREDIENTS

- 1 head cabbage, cored
- 4 tablespoons butter
- 2 tablespoons rendered bacon fat
- 1 chicken bouillon cube
- 1 teaspoon fresh ground black pepper
- 1garlic clove, minced.

DIRECTIONS

1. Preheat your smoker to 240 degrees Fahrenheit using your preferred wood
2. Fill the hole of your cored cabbage with butter, bouillon cube, bacon fat, pepper, and garlic
3. Wrap the cabbage in foil about two-thirds of the way up
4. Make sure to leave the top open
5. Transfer to your smoker rack and smoke for 2 hours
6. Unwrap and enjoy!

Nutritions: Calories: 231 Fats: 10g Carbs: 26g Fiber: 1g.

62. GARLIC AND ROSEMARY POTATO WEDGES

INGREDIENTS

- 4-6 large russet potatoes, cut into wedges
- ¼ cup olive oil
- 2garlic cloves, minced
- 2 tablespoons rosemary leaves, chopped
- 2 teaspoon salt
- 1 teaspoon fresh ground black pepper
- 1 teaspoon sugar
- 1 teaspoon onion powder.

DIRECTIONS

1. Preheat your smoker to 250 degrees Fahrenheit using maple wood.
2. Take a large bowl and add potatoes and olive oil.
3. Toss well.
4. Take another small bowl and stir garlic, salt, rosemary, pepper, sugar, onion powder.
5. Sprinkle the mix on all sides of the potato wedge.
6. Transfer the seasoned wedge to your smoker rack and smoke for 1 and a ½ hours.
7. Serve and enjoy!

Nutritions: Calories: 291 Fats: 10g Carbs: 46g Fiber: 2g.

63. SMOKED TOMATO AND MOZZARELLA DIP

INGREDIENTS

- 8 ounces smoked mozzarella cheese, shredded
- 8 ounces Colby cheese, shredded
- ½ cup parmesan cheese, grated
- 1 cup sour cream
- 1 cup sun-dried tomatoes
- 1 and ½ teaspoon salt
- 1 teaspoon fresh ground pepper
- 1 teaspoon dried basil
- 1 teaspoon dried oregano
- 1 teaspoon red pepper flakes
- 1garlic clove, minced
- ½ teaspoon onion powder
- French toast, serving.

DIRECTIONS

1. Preheat your smoker to 275 degrees Fahrenheit using your preferred wood
2. Take a large bowl and stir in the cheeses, tomatoes, pepper, salt, basil, oregano, red pepper flakes, garlic, onion powder and mix well
3. Transfer the mix to a small metal pan and transfer to a smoker
4. Smoke for 1 hour
5. Serve with toasted French bread
6. Enjoy!

Nutritions: Calories: 174 Fats: 11g Carbs: 15g Fiber: 2g.

CHAPTER 9. SEASONINGS AND SAUCES

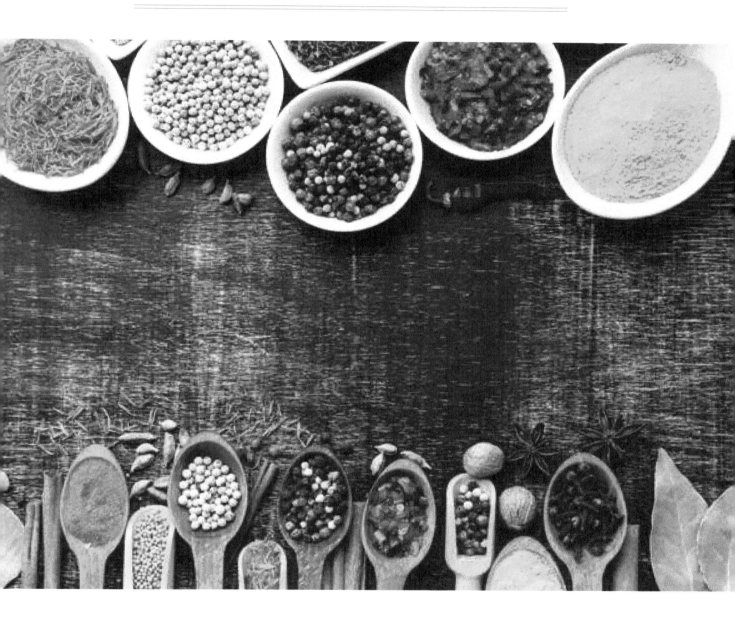

64. SMOKED TOMATO CREAM SAUCE

INGREDIENTS

- 1 lb. beefsteak tomatoes, fresh and quartered
- 1-1/2 tablespoon olive oil
- Black pepper, freshly ground
- Salt, kosher
- 1/2 cup yellow onions, chopped
- 1 tablespoon tomato paste
- 2 tablespoon minced garlic
- Pinch cayenne
- 1/2 cup chicken stock
- 1/2 cup heavy cream.

DIRECTIONS

1. Prepare your smoker using directions from the manufacturer.
2. Toss tomatoes and 1 tablespoon oil in a bowl, mixing, then season with pepper and salt.
3. Smoke the tomatoes placed on a smoker rack for about 30 minutes. Remove and set aside reserving tomato juices.
4. Heat 1/2 tablespoon oil in a saucepan over high-medium heat.
5. Add onion and cook for about 3-4 minutes. Add tomato paste and garlic, then cook for an additional 1 minute.
6. Add smoked tomatoes, cayenne, tomato juices, pepper, and salt, then cook for about 3-4 minutes. Stir often.
7. Add chicken stock and boil for about 25-30 minutes under a gentle simmer. Stir often.
8. Place the mixture in a blender and puree until smooth. Now squeeze the mixture through a sieve, fine mesh, to discard solids and release the juices,
9. Transfer the sauce to a saucepan, small, and add the cream.
10. Simmer for close to 6 minutes over low-medium heat until thickened slightly. Season with pepper and salt.
11. Serve warm with risotto cakes.

Nutritions: Calories: 50 Fat: 5g Carbohydrates: 2g Protein: 0g Fiber: 0g.

65. SMOKED MUSHROOM SAUCE

INGREDIENTS

- 1-quart chef mix mushrooms
- 2 tablespoon canola oil
- 1/4 cup julienned shallots
- 2 tablespoon chopped garlic
- Salt and pepper to taste
- 1/4 cup Alfasi Cabernet Sauvignon
- 1 cup beef stock
- 2 tablespoon margarine.

DIRECTIONS

1. Crumple four foil sheets into balls. Puncture multiple places in the foil pan, then place mushrooms in the foil pan. Smoke in a pellet grill for about 30 minutes. Remove and cool.
2. Heat canola oil in a pan, sauté, add shallots, and sauté until translucent.
3. Add mushrooms and cook until supple and rendered down.
4. Add garlic and season with pepper and salt. Cook until fragrant.
5. Add beef stock and wine, then cook for about 6-8 minutes over low heat. Adjust seasoning.
6. Add margarine and stir until sauce is thickened and a nice sheen.
7. Serve and enjoy!

Nutritions: Calories: 300 Fat: 30g Carbohydrates: 10g Protein: 4g Fiber: 0g.

66. SMOKED CRANBERRY SAUCE

INGREDIENTS

- 12 oz. bag cranberries
- 2 chunks ginger, quartered
- 1 cup apple cider
- 1 tablespoon honey whiskey
- 5.5 oz. fruit juice
- 1/8 tablespoon ground cloves
- 1/8 tablespoon cinnamon
- 1/2 orange zest
- 1/2 orange
- 1 tablespoon maple syrup
- 1 apple, diced and peeled
- 1/2 cup sugar
- 1/2 brown sugar.

DIRECTIONS

1. Preheat your pellet grill to 375°F.
2. Place cranberries in a pan, then add all other ingredients.
3. Place the pan on the grill and cook for about 1 hour until cooked through.
4. Remove ginger pieces and squeeze juices from the orange into the sauce.

Nutritions: Calories: 48 Total Fat: 0.1g Carbohydrates: 12.3g Protein: 0.4g Fiber: 2.3g.

67. SMOKED SRIRACHA SAUCE

INGREDIENTS

- 1 lb. Fresno chilies stems pulled off and seeds removed
- 1/2 cup rice vinegar
- 1/2 cup red wine vinegar
- 1 carrot, medium and cut into rounds, 1/4 inch
- 1-1/2 tablespoon sugar, dark brown
- 4garlic cloves, peeled
- 1 tablespoon olive oil
- 1 tablespoon kosher salt
- 1/2 cup water.

DIRECTIONS

1. Smoke chilies in a smoker for about 15 minutes.
2. Bring to boil both bottles of vinegar, then add carrots, sugar, and garlic. Simmer for about 15 minutes while covered. Cool for 30 minutes.
3. Place the chilies, olive oil, vinegar-vegetable mixture, salt, and ¼ cup water into a blender.
4. Blend for about 1-2 minutes on high. Add remaining water and blend again. You can add another 1/4 cup water if you want your sauce thinner.
5. Pour the sauce into jars and place them in a refrigerator.

Nutritions: Calories: 147 Fat: 5.23g Carbohydrates: 21g Protein: 3g Fiber: 3g.

68. SMOKED SOY SAUCE

INGREDIENTS

- 100ml soy sauce
- Bradley flavor Bisquettes Cherry.

DIRECTIONS

1. Put soy sauce in a heat-resistant bowl, large-mouth.
2. Smoke in a smoker at 158-176°F for about 1 hour. Stir a few times.
3. Remove and cool, then put in a bottle. Let sit for one day.
4. Serve and enjoy!

Nutritions: Calories: 110 Fat: 0g Carbohydrates: 25g Protein: 2g Fiber: 0g.

69. SMOKED GARLIC SAUCE

INGREDIENTS

- 3 whole garlic heads
- 1/2 cup mayonnaise
- 1/4 cup sour cream
- 2 tablespoon lemon juice
- 2 tablespoon cider vinegar
- Salt to taste.

DIRECTIONS

1. Cut the garlic heads off, then place in a microwave-safe bowl; add 2 tablespoon water and cover. Microwave for about 5-6 minutes on medium.
2. Heat your grill on medium.
3. Place the garlic heads in a shallow 'boat' foil and smoke for about 20-25 minutes until soft.
4. Transfer the garlic heads into a blender. Process for a few minutes until smooth.
5. Add remaining ingredients and process until everything is combined.

Nutritions: Calories: 20 Fat: 0g Carbohydrates: 10g Protein: 0g Fiber: 1g.

70. SMOKED CHERRY BARBECUE SAUCE

INGREDIENTS

- 2 lb. dark sweet cherries, pitted
- 1 large chopped onion
- 1/2 tablespoon red pepper flakes, crushed
- 1 tablespoon kosher salt or to taste
- 1/2 tablespoon ginger, ground
- 1/2 tablespoon black pepper
- 1/2 tablespoon cumin
- 1/2 tablespoon cayenne pepper
- 1 tablespoon onion powder
- 1 tablespoon garlic powder
- 1 tablespoon smoked paprika
- 2 chopped garlic cloves
- 1/2 cup pinot noir
- 2 tablespoon yellow mustard
- 1-1/2 cups ketchup
- 2 tablespoon balsamic vinegar
- 1/3 cup apple cider vinegar
- 2 tablespoon dark soy sauce
- 1 tablespoon liquid smoke
- 1/4 cup Worcestershire sauce
- 1 tablespoon hatch Chile powder
- 3 tablespoon honey
- 1 cup brown sugar
- 3 tablespoon molasses.

DIRECTIONS

1. Preheat your smoker to 250°F.
2. Place cherries in a baking dish, medium, and smoke for about 2 hours.
3. Sauté onions and red pepper flakes in a pot, large, with 2 tablespoon oil for about 4 minutes until softened.
4. Add salt and cook for an additional 1 minute.
5. Add ginger, black pepper, cumin, onion powder, garlic powder, and paprika, then drizzle with oil and cook for about 1 minute until fragrant and spices bloom.
6. Stir in garlic and cook for about 30 seconds.
7. Pour in pinot noir, scraping up for 1 minute for any bits stuck to your pan bottom.
8. Add yellow mustard, ketchup, balsamic vinegar, apple cider vinegar, dark soy sauce, liquid smoke, and Worcestershire sauce. Stir to combine.
9. Add cherries and simmer for about 10 minutes.
10. Add honey, brown sugar, and molasses and stir until combined. Simmer for about 30-45 minutes over low heat until your liking.
11. Place everything into a blender and process until a smooth sauce.
12. Enjoy with favorite veggies or protein. You can refrigerate in jars for up to a month.

Nutritions: Calories: 35 Fat: 0g Carbohydrates: 9g Protein: 0g Fiber: 0g.

71. SMOKED GARLIC WHITE SAUCE

INGREDIENTS

- 2 cups hickory wood chips, soaked in water for 30 minutes
- 3 whole garlic heads
- 1/2 cup mayonnaise
- 1/3 cup sour cream
- 1 juiced lemon
- 2 tablespoon apple cider vinegar
- Salt to taste.

DIRECTIONS

1. Cut garlic heads to expose the inside and place in a container, microwave-safe, with 2 tablespoon water. Microwave for about 5-6 minutes on medium.
2. Preheat your grill. Place garlic heads on a shallow foil "boat" and place it on the grill.
3. Close the grill and cook for about 20-25 minutes until soft completely. Remove and cool.
4. Transfer into a blender, then add the remaining ingredients. Process until smooth.
5. Serve immediately or store in a refrigerator for up to 5 days.

Nutritions: Calories: 20 Fat: 0g Carbohydrates: 8g Protein: 0g Fiber: 0g.

CHAPTER 10. DESSERTS

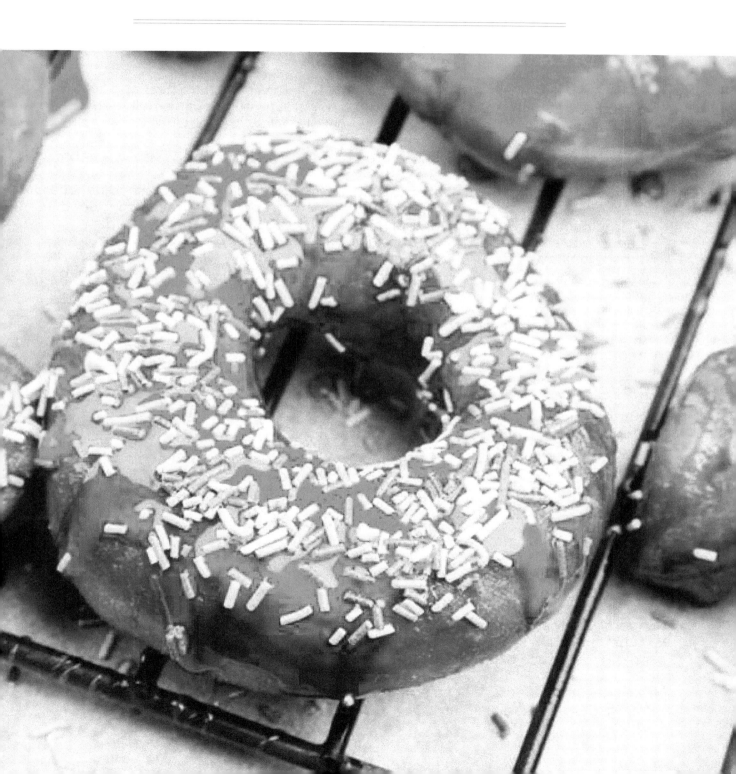

72. SMOKED BANANAS FOSTER BREAD PUDDING

INGREDIENTS

- 1 loaf (about 4 cups) brioche or challah, cubed into 1-inch cubes
- 3 eggs, lightly beaten
- 2 cups of milk
- 2/3 cups sugar
- 2 large bananas, peeled and smashed
- 1 tbsp. vanilla extract
- 1 tbsp. cinnamon
- 1/4 tsp. nutmeg
- 1/2 cup pecans.

Rum Sauce Ingredients:

- 1/2 cup spiced rum
- 1/4 cup unsalted butter
- 1 cup dark brown sugar
- 1 tsp. cinnamon
- 5 large bananas, peeled and quartered.

DIRECTIONS

1. Place pecans on a skillet over medium heat and lightly toast for about 5 minutes, until you can smell them.
2. Remove from heat and allow to cool. Once cooled, chop pecans.
3. Lightly butter a 9" x 13" baking dish and evenly layer bread cubes in the dish.
4. In a large bowl, whisk eggs, milk, sugar, mashed bananas, vanilla extract, cinnamon, and nutmeg until combined.
5. Pour egg mixture over the bread in the baking dish evenly. Sprinkle with chopped pecans. Cover with aluminum foil and refrigerate for about 30 minutes.
6. Preheat pellet grill to 180°F. Turn your smoke setting to high, if applicable.
7. Remove foil from dish and place on the smoker for 5 minutes with the lid closed, allowing bread to absorb smoky flavor.
8. Remove dish from the grill and cover with foil again. Increase your pellet grill's temperature to 350°F.
9. Place dish on the grill grate and cook for 50-60 minutes until everything is cooked through and the bread pudding is bubbling.
10. In a saucepan, while pudding cooks, heat up butter for rum sauce over medium heat. When the butter begins to melt, add the brown sugar, cinnamon, and bananas. Sauté until bananas begin to soften.
11. Add rum and watch. When the liquid begins to bubble, light a match, and tilt the pan. Slowly and carefully move the match towards the liquid until the sauce lights. When the flames go away, remove skillet from heat.
12. If you're uncomfortable lighting the liquid with a match, just cook it for 3-4 minutes over medium heat after the rum has been added.
13. Keep rum sauce on a simmer or reheat once it's time to serve.
14. Remove bread pudding from the grill and allow it to cool for about 5 minutes.
15. Cut into squares, put each square on a plate and add a piece of banana, then drizzle rum sauce over the top. Serve on its own or a la mode and enjoy it!

Nutritions: Calories: 274.7 Fat: 7.9g Cholesterol: 10mg Carbohydrates: 35.5g Fiber: 0.9gSugar: 24.7g Protein: 4g.

73. GRILLED POUND CAKE WITH FRUIT DRESSING

INGREDIENTS

- 1 buttermilk pound cake, sliced into 3/4 inch slices
- 1/8 cup butter, melted
- 1.1/2 cup whipped cream
- 1/2 cup blueberries
- 1/2 cup raspberries
- 1/2 cup strawberries, sliced.

DIRECTIONS

1. Preheat pellet grill to 400°F. Turn your smoke setting to high, if applicable.
2. Brush both sides of each pound cake slice with melted butter.
3. Place directly on the grill grate and cook for 5 minutes per side. Turn 90° halfway through cooking each side of the cake for checkered grill marks.
4. You can cook a couple of minutes longer if you prefer deeper grill marks and smoky flavor.
5. Remove pound cake slices from the grill and allow it to cool on a plate.
6. Top slices with whipped cream, blueberries, raspberries, and sliced strawberries as desired. Serve and enjoy!

Nutritions: Calories: 222.1 Fat: 8.7g Cholesterol: 64.7mg Carbohydrates: 33.1g Fiber: 0.4g Sugar: 20.6g Protein: 3.4g.

74. GRILLED PINEAPPLE WITH CHOCOLATE SAUCE

INGREDIENTS

- 1 pineapple
- 8 oz. bittersweet chocolate chips
- 1/2 cup spiced rum
- 1/2 cup whipping cream
- 2 tbsp. light brown sugar.

DIRECTIONS

1. Preheat pellet grill to 400°F.
2. De-skin the pineapple and slice pineapple into 1 in cubes.
3. In a saucepan, combine chocolate chips. When chips begin to melt, add rum to the saucepan. Continue to stir until combined, then add a splash of the pineapple's juice.
4. Add in whipping cream and continue to stir the mixture. Once the sauce is smooth and thickening, lower heat to simmer to keep warm.
5. Thread pineapple cubes onto skewers. Sprinkle skewers with brown sugar.
6. Place skewers on the grill grate. Grill for about 5 minutes per side, or until grill marks begin to develop.
7. Remove skewers from grill and allow to rest on a plate for about 5 minutes. Serve alongside warm chocolate sauce for dipping.

Nutritions: Calories: 112.6 Fat: 0.5g Cholesterol: 0 Carbohydrates: 28.8g Fiber: 1.6g Sugar: 0.1g Protein: 0.4g.

75. NECTARINE AND NUTELLA SUNDAE

INGREDIENTS

- 2 nectarines, halved and pitted
- 2 tsp. honey
- 4 tbsp. Nutella
- 4 scoops vanilla ice cream
- 1/4 cup pecans, chopped
- Whipped cream, to top
- 4 cherries, to top.

DIRECTIONS

1. Preheat pellet grill to 400°F.
2. Slice nectarines in half and remove the pits.
3. Brush the inside (cut side) of each nectarine half with honey.
4. Place nectarines directly on the grill grate, cut side down. Cook for 5-6 minutes, or until grill marks develop.
5. Flip nectarines and cook on the other side for about 2 minutes.
6. Remove nectarines from the grill and allow it to cool.
7. Fill the pit cavity on each nectarine half with 1 tbsp. Nutella.
8. Place 1 scoop of ice cream on top of Nutella. Top with whipped cream, cherries, and sprinkle chopped pecans. Serve and enjoy!

Nutritions: Calories: 90 Fat: 3g Cholesterol: 0 Carbohydrates: 15g Fiber: 0 Sugar: 13g Protein: 2g.

76. CINNAMON SUGAR DONUT HOLES

INGREDIENTS

- 1/2 cup flour
- 1 tbsp. cornstarch
- 1/2 tsp. baking powder
- 1/8 tsp. baking soda
- 1/8 tsp. ground cinnamon
- 1/2 tsp. kosher salt
- 1/4 cup buttermilk
- 1/4 cup sugar
- 1 1/2 tbsp. butter, melted
- 1 egg
- 1/2 tsp. vanilla

Topping:

- 2tbsp. sugar
- 1tbsp. sugar
- 1tsp. ground cinnamon.

DIRECTIONS

1. Preheat pellet grill to 350°F.
2. In a medium bowl, combine flour, cornstarch, baking powder, baking soda, ground cinnamon, and kosher salt. Whisk to combine.
3. In a separate bowl, combine buttermilk, sugar, melted butter, egg, and vanilla. Whisk until the egg is thoroughly combined.
4. Pour wet mixture into the flour mixture and stir. Stir just until combined, careful not to overwork the mixture.
5. Spray mini muffin tin with cooking spray.
6. Spoon 1 tbsp. of donut mixture into each mini muffin hole.
7. Place the tin on the pellet grill grate and bake for about 18 minutes, or until a toothpick can come out clean.
8. Remove muffin tin from the grill and let rest for about 5 minutes.
9. In a small bowl, combine 1 tbsp. sugar and 1 tsp. ground cinnamon.
10. Melt 2 tbsp. of butter in a glass dish. Dip each donut hole in the melted butter, then mix and toss with cinnamon sugar. Place completed donut holes on a plate to serve.

Nutritions: Calories: 190 Fat: 17g Cholesterol: 0 Carbohydrates: 21g Fiber: 1g Sugar: 8g Protein: 3g.

77. PELLET GRILL CHOCOLATE CHIP COOKIES

INGREDIENTS

- 1 cup salted butter softened
- 1 cup of sugar
- 1 cup light brown sugar
- 2 tsp. vanilla extract
- 2 large eggs
- 3cups all-purpose flour
- 1 tsp. baking soda
- 1/2 tsp. baking powder
- 1 tsp. natural sea salt
- 2 cups semi-sweet chocolate chips or chunks.

DIRECTIONS

1. Preheat pellet grill to 375°F.
2. Line a large baking sheet with parchment paper and set aside.
3. In a medium bowl, mix flour, baking soda, salt, and baking powder. Once combined, set aside.
4. In stand mixer bowl, combine butter, white sugar, and brown sugar until combined. Beat in eggs and vanilla. Beat until fluffy.
5. Mix in dry ingredients, continue to stir until combined.
6. Add chocolate chips and mix thoroughly.
7. Roll 3 tbsp. of dough at a time into balls and place them on your cookie sheet. Evenly space them apart, with about 2-3 inches in between each ball.
8. Place cookie sheet directly on the grill grate and bake for 20-25 minutes, until the outside of the cookies is slightly browned.
9. Remove from grill and allow to rest for 10 minutes. Serve and enjoy!

Nutritions: Calories: 120 Fat: 4 Cholesterol: 7.8mg Carbohydrates: 22.8g Fiber: 0.3g Sugar: 14.4g Protein: 1.4g.

78. DELICIOUS DONUTS ON A GRILL

INGREDIENTS

- 1-1/2 cups sugar, powdered
- 1/3 cup whole milk
- 1/2 teaspoon vanilla extract
- 16 ounces of biscuit dough, prepared
- Oil spray, for greasing
- 1 cup chocolate sprinkles for sprinkling.

DIRECTIONS

1. Take a medium bowl and mix sugar, milk, and vanilla extract.
2. Combine well to create a glaze.
3. Set the glaze aside for further use.
4. Place the dough onto the flat, clean surface.
5. Flat the dough with a rolling pin.
6. Use a ring mold, about an inch, and cut the hole in the center of each round dough.
7. Place the dough on a plate and refrigerate for 10 minutes.
8. Open the grill and install the grill grate inside it.
9. Close the hood.
10. Now, select the grill from the menu, and set the temperature to medium.
11. Set the time to 6 minutes.
12. Select start and begin preheating.
13. Remove the dough from the refrigerator and coat it with cooking spray from both sides.
14. When the unit beeps, the grill is preheated; place the adjustable amount of dough on the grill grate.
15. Close the hood, and cook for 3 minutes.
16. After 3 minutes, remove donuts and place the remaining dough inside.
17. Cook for 3 minutes.
18. Once all the donuts are ready, sprinkle chocolate sprinkles on top.
19. Enjoy.

Nutritions: Calories: 400 Total Fat: 11g Saturated Fat: 4.2g Cholesterol: 1mg Sodium: 787mg Total Carbohydrates: 71.3g Dietary Fiber: 0.9g Total Sugars: 45.3g Protein: 5.7g.

79. SMOKED PUMPKIN PIE

INGREDIENTS

- 1 tbsp. cinnamon
- 1-1/2 tbsp. pumpkin pie spice
- 15 oz. can pumpkin
- 14 oz. can sweetened condensed milk
- 2 beaten eggs
- 1 unbaked pie shell
- Topping: whipped cream.

DIRECTIONS

1. Preheat your smoker to 325°F.
2. Place a baking sheet, rimmed, on the smoker upside down, or use a cake pan.
3. Combine all your ingredients in a bowl, large, except the pie shell, then pour the mixture into a pie crust.
4. Place the pie on the baking sheet and smoke for about 50-60 minutes until a knife comes out clean when inserted. Make sure the center is set.
5. Remove and cool for about 2 hours or refrigerate overnight.
6. Serve with a whipped cream dollop and enjoy it!

Nutritions: Calories: 292 Total Fat: 11g Saturated Fat: 5g Total Carbs: 42g Net Carbs: 40g Protein: 7g Sugars: 29g Fiber: 5g Sodium: 168mg.

80. WOOD PELLET SMOKED NUT MIX

INGREDIENTS

- 3 cups mixed nuts (pecans, peanuts, almonds, etc.)
- 1/2 tbsp. brown sugar
- 1 tbsp. thyme, dried
- 1/4 tbsp. mustard powder
- 1 tbsp. olive oil, extra-virgin.

DIRECTIONS

1. Preheat your pellet grill to 250°F with the lid closed for about 15 minutes.
2. Combine all ingredients in a bowl, large, then transfer into a cookie sheet lined with parchment paper.
3. Place the cookie sheet on a grill and grill for about 20 minutes.
4. Remove the nuts from the grill and let cool.
5. Serve and enjoy.

Nutritions: Calories: 249 Total Fat: 21.5g Saturated Fat: 3.5g Total Carbs: 12.3g Net Carbs: 10.1g Protein: 5.7g Sugars: 5.6g Fiber: 2.1g Sodium: 111mg.

81. GRILLED PEACHES AND CREAM

INGREDIENTS

- 4 halved and pitted peaches
- 1 tbsp. vegetable oil
- 2 tbsp. clover honey
- 1 cup cream cheese, soft with honey and nuts.

DIRECTIONS

1. Preheat your pellet grill to medium-high heat.
2. Coat the peaches lightly with oil and place on the grill pit side down.
3. Grill for about 5 minutes until nice grill marks on the surfaces.
4. Turn over the peaches, then drizzle with honey.
5. Spread and cream cheese dollop where the pit was and grill for additional 2-3 minutes until the filling becomes warm.
6. Serve immediately.

Nutritions: Calories: 139 Total Fat: 10.2g Saturated Fat: 5g Total Carbs: 11.6g Net Carbs: 11.6g Protein: 1.1g Sugars: 12g Fiber: 0g Sodium: 135mg.

82. BERRY COBBLER ON A PELLET GRILL

INGREDIENTS

For the fruit filling:

- 3cups frozen mixed berries
- 1lemon juice
- 1cup brown sugar
- 1tbsp. vanilla extract
- 1bsp lemon zest, finely grated.
- A pinch of salt.

For cobbler topping:

- 1-1/2 cups all-purpose flour
- 1-1/2 tbsp. baking powder
- 3 tbsp. sugar, granulated
- 1/2 tbsp. salt
- 8 tbsp. cold butter
- 1/2 cup sour cream
- 2 tbsp. raw sugar.

DIRECTIONS

1. Set your pellet grill on "smoke" for about 4-5 minutes with the lid open until fire establishes, and your grill starts smoking.
2. Preheat your grill to 350°F for about 10-15 minutes with the grill lid closed.
3. Meanwhile, combine frozen mixed berries, Lemon juice, brown sugar, vanilla, lemon zest, and a pinch of salt. Transfer into a skillet and let the fruit sit and thaw.
4. Mix flour, baking powder, sugar, and salt in a bowl, medium. Cut cold butter into peas sizes using a pastry blender, then add to the mixture. Stir to mix everything.
5. Stir in sour cream until dough starts coming together.
6. Pinch small pieces of dough and place over the fruit until fully covered. Splash the top with raw sugar.
7. Now place the skillet directly on the grill grate, close the lid and cook for about 35 minutes until juices bubble and a golden-brown dough topping.
8. Remove the skillet from the pellet grill and cool for several minutes.
9. Scoop and serve warm.

Nutritions: Calories: 371 Total Fat: 13g Saturated Fat: 8g Total Carbs: 60g Net Carbs: 58g Protein: 3g Sugars: 39g Fiber: 2g Sodium: 269mg.

83. PELLET GRILL APPLE CRISP

INGREDIENTS

Apples:

- 10 large apples
- 1/2 cup flour
- 1cup sugar, dark brown
- 1/2 tbsp. cinnamon
- 1/2 cup butter slices.

Crisp:

- 3 cups oatmeal, old-fashioned
- 1-1/2 cups softened butter, salted
- 1-1/2 tbsp. cinnamon
- 2 cups brown sugar.

DIRECTIONS

1. Preheat your grill to 350°F.
2. Wash, peel, core, and dice the apples into cubes, medium-size
3. Mix flour, dark brown sugar, and cinnamon, then toss with your apple cubes.
4. Spray a baking pan, 10x13", with cooking spray, then place apples inside. Top with butter slices.
5. Mix all crisp ingredients in a medium bowl until well combined. Place the mixture over the apples.
6. Place on the grill and cook for about 1-hour checking after every 15-20 minutes to ensure cooking is even. Do not place it on the hottest grill part.
7. Remove and let sit for about 20-25 minutes
8. It's very warm.

Nutritions: Calories: 528 Total Fat: 26g Saturated Fat: 16g Total Carbs: 75g Net Carbs: 70g Protein: 4g Sugars: 51g Fiber: 5g Sodium: 209mg.

84. SMOKED PEACH PARFAIT

INGREDIENTS

- 4 barely ripe peaches halved and pitted
- 1 tablespoon firmly packed brown sugar
- 1 pint vanilla ice cream
- 3 tablespoons honey.

DIRECTIONS

1. Preheat your smoker to 200 degrees Fahrenheit
2. Sprinkle cut peach halves with brown sugar
3. Transfer them to smoker and smoke for 33-45 minutes
4. Transfer the peach halves to dessert plates and top with vanilla ice cream
5. Drizzle honey and serve!

Nutritions: Calories: 309 Fats: 27g Carbs: 17g Fiber: 2g.

85. GRILLED FRUIT AND CREAM

INGREDIENTS

- 2 apricots, halved
- 1 nectarine, halved
- 2 peaches, halved
- ¼ cup blueberries
- ½ cup raspberries
- 2 tablespoons honey
- 1 orange, peel
- 2 cups cream
- ½ cup balsamic vinegar.

DIRECTIONS

1. Preheat your smoker to 400 degrees F, lid closed
2. Grill peaches, nectarines, apricots for 4 minutes, each side
3. Place pan on the stove and turn on medium heat
4. Add 2 tablespoons honey, vinegar, orange peel
5. Simmer until medium-thick
6. Add honey and cream in a bowl and whip until it reaches a soft form
7. Place fruits on serving plate and sprinkle berries, drizzle balsamic reduction
8. Serve with cream and enjoy!

Nutritions: Calories: 230 Fats: 3g Carbs: 35g Fiber: 2g.

86. APPLE PIE GRILL

INGREDIENTS

- ¼ cup of sugar
- 4 apples, sliced
- 1 tablespoon cornstarch
- 1 teaspoon cinnamon, ground
- 1 pie crust, refrigerator, soften in according to the directions on the box
- ½ cup peach preserves.

DIRECTIONS

1. Preheat your smoker to 375 degrees F, the closed lid
2. Take a bowl and add cinnamon, cornstarch, apples and keep it on the side
3. Place piecrust in pie pan and spread preserves, place apples
4. Fold crust slightly
5. Place pan on your smoker (upside down), smoke for 30-40 minutes
6. Once done, let it rest
7. Serve and enjoy!

Nutritions: Calories: 160 Fats: 1g Carbs: 35g Fiber: 1g.

CONCLUSION

Pellet grills are revolutionary and may forever change the way we cook.

These days, anyone can own a pellet grill since manufacturers meet the demand of clients from various backgrounds.

Modern pellet grills make cooking enjoyable and hassle-free.

It also eliminates guesswork thanks to the easy-to-follow recipes and the ability to remotely monitor and adjust your temperatures.

Whether you're an amateur home cook hosting a backyard cookout or a pitmaster at a barbecue competition, a wood pellet grill can easily become one of the most important appliances you can own to help you make flavorful meals with much less effort.

Although wood pellets grill isn't everyone's favorite choice, it's clear that a wood pellet grill is a must-have outdoor kitchen appliance. Whether you love smoking, grilling, roasting, barbecuing, or direct cooking of food, the wood pellet grill is clearly versatile and has got you covered.

Cooking with a wood pellet grill allows you to choose the desired flavor of wood pellets to create the perfect smoke to flavor your food. Each wood pellet type has its personality and taste. The best part is you can use a single flavor or experiment with mixing and matching the flavors to invent your own combination.

Just like any cooking appliance, wood pellets have some drawbacks, but the benefits overshadow them. It is, therefore, definitely worth a try.

These days, one popular method of cooking is smoking, which many enthusiasts use. Proteins such as different kinds of meat, poultry, and fish would be ruined quickly if modern techniques in cooking are used. Smoking, on the other hand, is a process that takes a long time and low temperature, which thoroughly cooks the meat. The smoke, especially white smoke, greatly enhances the flavor of almost any food item. But more than that, smoking seals and preserves the nutrients in the food. Smoking is flexible and is one of the oldest techniques for making food.

Someone once dubbed smoking as a form of art. Only with a minimal period of consistent effort, any enthusiast can easily master the basics and advanced techniques. It is even said that once you master and improve on your expertise in smoking, you will not consider the other techniques in cooking to master anymore. But because of the many smoking techniques, you have to find a technique that is suitable for your temperament and style. You can do that by experimentation and trials of different smoking methods and different kinds of woods. Try cooking meat products for several hours using a heat source, not directly on the meat. But you have to make sure that the smoke has a space to soak your meat and give it an access way out.

The picture of a good time with loved ones, neighbors, and friends having a backyard barbeque is a pretty sight, isn't it? Having a smoker-grill and some grilled and smoked recipes are excellent when you have visitors at home because you can deliver both tasty food and magical moment on a summer night, for example. Hundreds of awesome recipes are available that you can try with a wood pellet smoker-grill! Experiment, improve, or make your own recipes – it is up to you. You can do it fast and easy. But if you want to be safe with the proven and tested ones, by all means do it. These recipes have been known to be just right to the taste, and they work every time. A combination of creating a correct impression the first time and every time and enjoying scrumptious food along the way will be your edge.

Another great thing about these recipes is that they are easy to prepare and do not require you to be a wizard in the kitchen. Simply by following a few easy steps and having the right ingredients at your disposal, you can use these recipes to make some delicious food in no time. So, try these recipes and spread the word! I'm sure this wood pellet smoker-grill recipe book will prove to be an invaluable gift to your loved ones, too!

Finally, while you will have fantastic smoking and grilling time with whichever wood pellet grill model you choose, the models are quite different. They hence offer different services and are suitable for different users. With new wood pellet grill series being produced each year, you need to shop smart so that you buy a grill that perfectly fits you and meets all your needs.

If you are considering buying a grill yourself, then first you need to know the best kind of grills out in the market and what will suit you. You need to know how they work, compare, and which ones are trending. Traeger wood pellet grill is top on the markets and has many advantages over the standard cooking grill everyone has. New technology is coming out with better and better products to choose from, and if you don't upgrade your purchase and keep buying the same old stuff, then you will be left behind.

The Traeger grill provides a person which a great barbecuing experience with everyone, making food tastes better and cooking easier.

Now you no longer have to scour the web, hunting for your favorite wood pellet smoker-grill recipes. This book is a one-stop solution designed to eliminate all your struggles in finding the perfect wood pellet smoker-grill recipes for yourself and your loved ones.

CPSIA information can be obtained
at www.ICGtesting.com
Printed in the USA
LVHW060317230221
679613LV00006B/252